The Inflammatory and Atresia-Inducing Disease of the Liver and Bile Ducts

Monographs in Paediatrics

Vol. 8

S. Karger · Basel · München · Paris · London · New York · Sydney

The Inflammatory and Atresia-Inducing Disease of the Liver and Bile Ducts

A. Pérez-Soler

Professor of Paediatrics, Autonomous University of Barcelona

With 17 figures, 16 color plates and 11 tables, 1976

S. Karger · Basel · München · Paris · London · New York · Sydney

Monographs in Paediatrics

Previously published

Vo. 1–3: please ask for details.
Vol. 4: KLAUS A. ZUPPINGER (Bern): Hypoglycemia in Childhood. Evaluation of Diagnostic Procedures.
VI + 135 p., 34 fig., 42 tab., 1975. ISBN 3-8055-2061-1.
Vol. 5: E. E. JOSS (Bern): Growth Hormone Deficiency in Childhood. Evaluation of Diagnostic Procedures.
VIII + 83 p., 33 fig., 10 tab., 1975. ISBN 3-8055-2159-6.
Vol. 6: PAUL R. SWYER (Toronto, Ontario). With a contribution by M. ANN LLEWELLYN (Toronto, Ontario): The Intensive Care of the Newly Born. Physiological Principles and Practice.
X + 208 p., 45 fig., 35 tab., 1975. ISBN 3-8055-2184-7.
Vol. 7: ROLF P. ZURBRÜGG (Biel): Hypothalamic-Pituitary-Adrenocortical (HPA) Regulation. A Contribution to Its Assessment, Development and Disorders in Infancy and Childhood with Special Reference to Plasma Cortisol Circadian Rhythm.
VIII + 83 p., 49 fig., 14 tab., 1976. ISBN 3-8055-2253-3.

Cataloging in Publication
Pérez-Soler, A.
The inflammatory and atresia-inducing disease of the liver and bile ducts/A. Pérez-Soler. – Basel; New York: Karger, 1976.
(Monographs in paediatrics; v. 8)
1. Bile Ducts, Intrahepatic – abnormalities 2. Bile Ducts – abnormalities 3. Hepatitis – in infancy & childhood I. Title II. Series
W1 MO568G v. 8/WI 700 P439i
ISBN 3-8055-2257-6

Contents

Contents

The Triad
Extrahepatic Biliary Atresia
Neonatal Hepatitis and
Intrahepatic Biliary Atresia
a Pathogenic Unit:

The Inflammatory and Atresia-Inducing
Disease of the Liver and Bile Ducts

To my father
who, in spite of his humble condition,
communicated to me
the interest for everything
and stimulated my heuristic spirit.

Introduction

Extrahepatic biliary atresia, neonatal hepatitis, and intrahepatic biliary atresia are three diseases that have been known for a long time and which have become increasingly important in the practice of pediatrics; they are included in the extensive and complex chapter on 'Neonatal jaundice prolonged into infancy' and in the subgroup on 'Jaundice with predominance of direct hyperbilirubinemia'.

It is well known that the etiology of these entities remains to be proved. In relation to atresias, even today the majority of authors admit a genetic alteration at the gene level that would fit pathogenically into the classic conception of agenesia. By 'neonatal hepatitis', we refer specifically to the hepatitis with giant cell transformation, which constitutes one of the most outstanding diseases in the complex and variegated field of neonatal hepatitis; the general consensus is that the process responds to an acquired etiology. A good number of authors, basing their conclusions on epidemiological data and on the patho-clinical characteristics, favor a viral cause.

It is true that these etiological theories have, until very recently, been little more than scantily documented surmises. Nevertheless, the discovery by COLE et al. of the hepatitis virus in some cases of 'neonatal hepatitis' and in one case of atresia, the recent demonstration by STRAUSS and BERNSTEIN that the rubella virus can produce the ductal lessions usually found in atresia, and the recent communication by TOLENTINO et al. about two cases of partial intrahepatic atresia and extrabiliary agenesia with the presence of the Australia antigen (HAA) in the children and in their mothers (who had not shown any symptoms during pregnancy and did not have any previous history of hepatitis), all seem to cast a brilliant light on the etiology of such diseases. This will stimulate pediatricians to prod researchers in virology to consider with utmost attention and as a question of their own this exciting pediatric problem.

The interest on the knowledge of the entities of this *triad,* i.e. extrahepatic biliary atresia, neonatal hepatitis, and intrahepatic biliary atresia, is enhanced by the fact that they seem to have remarkably increased in the last decades. Has this to do with the 'pathomorphosis' undergone by viral hepatitis, which has become more frequent? We believe it is very likely.

Up to now, most authors concerned about these entities have considered them as independent. More particularly, extrahepatic biliary atresia and neonatal hepatitis have been assumed to be separate entities related only from a clinical point of view, due to some common signs, especially from the standpoint of jaundice, which physiopathologically corresponds to a deficiency in the excretion of bile. But both are pathogenically very different: *atresia is attributed to a disorder of embryonic development and hepatitis to an inflammatory process.* Intrahepatic biliary atresia, whose icteric sign responds to the same physiopathology, has already been considered less independent, and nearly always involved with only one of them. In fact, the vast majority of authors consider it within extrahepatic biliary atresia, simply because it often coincides with the latter.

Is this really so? Is it certain that the most outstanding feature of the 'link' between these entities is their jaundice by 'regurgitation' and that there exists no pathogenic relation between atresia and hepatitis?

We base our conception on a good number of observations: The great majority with definitive diagnosis confirmed by necropsy, or prolonged catamnesis, and some of them observed for many years, which we have had the chance to study in the Pediatric Surgical Department of Dr. E. ROVIRALTA and in the Pediatric Clinic for Infectious Diseases of Dr. SALA GINABREDA in Barcelona and those of other colleagues we have been allowed to check or supervise; these observations are distributed as follows:

	Cases
Extrahepatic atresia	12
Intrahepatic atresia	4
Intrahepatic atresia of the large ducts near the hilum	1
Neonatal hepatitis	9
Total	26

Other observations are being studied by special biologic analysis (investigation of hepatitis-associated antigens, determination of isoenzymes of alkaline phosphatase, a_1-antitrypsin, etc.); several observations carried out in the University Pediatric Clinic of the Faculty of Medicine of Montpellier whose histological studies we have been able to check; and the study of special cases of jaundice in the young infant, among them two with MacMahon-Thannhauser syndrome which appeared in early infancy born to consanguineous parents in two brothers and another, a family case, with acute atrophy of the liver secondary to viral hepatitis. All this material and the consultation of a vast bibliography has led us to believe that *the three diseases constitute a single unit from a pathogenic point of view*. A good number of patho-clinical facts support this suggestion.

We do not pretend our studies to be exhaustive, although they are necessarily extensive on account of the great importance and complexity of the subject. We think that it is indispensable to include the points of view of a good number of authors who have been concerned with these three entities. The problem which can still only be speculated upon in many fields, especially the nosological, has unwittingly lengthened our task. The book has been printed in two different type sizes. The main parts of the text give a panoramic view of the problem; for more detail, read the paragraphs printed in petit characters.

We do not intend to dogmatize or to establish definitive conclusions. If we put forward and defend this unitarian pathogenic theory, it is, moreover, with the intention of fitting in one of the entities which is considered to be 'separate', the intrahepatic biliary atresia, viewed as little less than a 'confusing element', which came to complicate the clinical diagnostical maze which existed between the two entities and which the modern means of analytical research has not yet completely solved.

We are convinced that this unipathogenic view of the diseases included in the *triad* has a greater aim than a simple desire for a synthesis. We believe it will help towards a better nosological understanding of them from which more soundly based therapeutical measures will be developed.

We believe that certain viewpoints will be subject to debate and even some of them might be rejected. Nevertheless, if our work may be of use for others to find, above all, the solution to the etiological and therapeutical problems of these diseases, we will consider to have succeeded in our goal.

Finally, we must express our sincere and lasting gratitude to all those who have helped and advised us in the production of this work. Most especially we would like to recognize our debt to the Drs. E. ROVIRALTA and J. M. SALA GINABREDA, directors of the departments in which we have carried out the majority of our observations, and to the principal collaborator of the latter, Dr. J. LLORENS TEROL. We express our gratitude to Dr. L. GUBERN SALISACHS with whom a great cooperation has existed in the study of various observations and particularly for having considered with singular attention our points of view over a sphere in which he has penetrated so deeply, and to the professors of Montpellier, R. JEAN and A. PAGÉS. We extend our gratitude to other colleagues who have allowed us to check or supervise their observations, especially to Drs. M. CARBONELL JUANICO, J. PICAÑOL, J. MARTÍNEZ MORA, and G. FIGUERAS from Barcelona, and to the Zaragoza colleagues, Prof. M. TABUENCA, Drs. L. BONÉ SANDOVAL, and A. PUEYO GARCÍA. We acknowledge the cooperation of the pathologists E. CAÑADAS SAURAS, J. RUBIÓ ROIG, and A. NOGUERA MUEDRA; of the biochemist Prof. Dr. A. COROMINAS VILARDELL and of the Prof. of Biometry and Statistics, Dr. A. FONTDEVILA VIVANCO. Dr. J. VIVES MAÑÉ deserves a particular mention for his excellent technical knowledge on microphotography.

The printing of this book has been possible thanks to the financial help of the following pharmaceutical Divisions: Antibioticos S. A.; Baldacci Prod. (Dypsa); Böhringer Sohn, S. A. E., Ingelheim; Lasa Laboratories; Lederle (Cyanamid Ib); Menarini S. A.; Merck-Igoda S. A.; Milupa S. A.; Novofarma S. A.; Schering Corp. (Essex S. A.); and Wander S. A. E.

Chapter 1

Clinical Signs and Laboratory Findings

Extrahepatic biliary atresia, neonatal hepatitis, and intrahepatic biliary atresia, each offer the picture of an icteric syndrome with very similar clinical and biological aspects, practically identical on many occasions and which are being mentioned repeatedly in the literature. This is the reason why, with the intention of not indulging in unnecessary repetitions, and with the leitmotiv of our work in sight, we are going to consider jointly the three entities from the clinical standpoint, describing and discussing their most important clinical features and indicating especially the analytic signs and tests which are considered of value for their differential diagnosis.

The position of the three entities in the extensive group of neonatal jaundice prolonged into infancy is indicated in the following list.

I. Neonatal Jaundice Prolonged into Infancy

A. Clinical-Pathogenic-Etiological Classification

A. Physiological
Simple transitory jaundice of the newborn which can occasionally be pathologic in: prematurity and fetal dystrophy

B. Pathological
1. Hemolytic
   a. Isoimmunization
      Rh
      ABO
      Others

      b. Hemoglobinosis (hereditary disorder in the synthesis of hemoglobin)
         Thalassemia
         Sickle cell anemia
         Others
      c. Erythrocytic genodystrophies
         1) Spherocytosis
            a) Hereditary (Minkowsky-Chauffard)
            b) Nonhereditary
         2) With enzymatic defect (enzymopenic erithropathy)
            a) Known types
               Glucose-6-phosphate dehydrogenase
               Piruvate-kinase
               Dyphosphate-glyceromutase, etc.
            b) Still unidentified
      d. Increased hemolysis due to extensive hematomata
      e. Due to other hemolyzing causes
         Toxic
         Drug-induced, etc.

2. Primarily dysmetabolic (due to enzymatic defects of the liver cell)
      a. Congenital
         1) As isolated hepatic disease
            a) Due to a deficit in the conjugation of bilirubin
               Exclusive
                   Accidental: 'physiological' jaundice of the premature or of the fetal
                   dystrophy
                   As an inborn enzymatic error: Crigler-Najjar disease
                   Associated to a deficit in the uptake of indirect bilirubin by the liver cell:
                   Gilbert disease (familial cholemia)
            b) Due to a difficulty
               Of intracellular transport of the conjugated bilirubin?
               Of the excretion through the membrane:
                   Dublin-Johnson disease
                   Rotor disease
         2) In other congenital diseases where one or various of the forementioned
            dysenzymatic causes may be present
               Congenital myxedema
               Mongolism
               Galactosemia
               Thirosinemia
               Ornitinemia
               Piloric stenosis, etc.
      b. Acquired
         Various enzymatic inhibition by intoxications
         Inhibition of the glucorinization by a factor in mother's milk

3. Primarily inflammatory

    a. Common, simple jaundice, due to infections by:
       Syphilis
       Toxoplasmosis
       Hepatitis virus A and B
       Herpes virus
       Cytomegalia
       Rubella virus
       Coxsackie virus
       Bacterial sepsis, etc.
    b. *Inflammatory and atresia-inducing disease* of the liver and bile ducts. Viral etiology very likely in the majority of cases. Fetopathy with three possible clinical-pathological expressions:
       Extrahepatic biliary atresia
       Neonatal hepatitis
       Intrahepatic biliary atresia

4. Congenital fibro-cirrhotic. Diseases that can occasionally cause jaundice at birth or shortly afterwards
       Familial fibrosis or cirrhosis
       Cirrhosis due to mucoviscidosis
       Fibrosis and cirrhosis of diverse etiologies, many of them attributed to the hepatitis virus

5. True malformations of the bile ducts. Dysgenesic or agenesic as an expression of blastopathy or embriopathy, due to a genic anomaly or acquired noxae during the preembryonic or embryonic period
    a. Limited to the ducts
       Some exceptional cases of biliary atresia?
       Fibroangiomatosis of the intrahepatic ducts
    b. Associated with malformations in other organs
       e.g. In the kidney (fibroangiomatosis of the intrahepatic ducts associated to a renal tubular dilation)

6. Intrahepatic obstructive. Diseases of known or unknown etiology in which the obstruction of the intrahepatic ducts is relevant
       By tumoral elements that obstruct preferentially the ducts near the hilum
       By thrombus of cytomegalic inclusion cells
       Inspissated bile syndrome?

7. Obstructive of the external bile ducts
    a. Due to intrinsic causes
       Common bile duct cyst
       Gallbladder anomaly: joined to the duodenum, but not by the common bile duct
       Pathological products: mucous plugs in some cases of mucoviscidosis, etc.
    b. Due to extrinsic causes
       Compression by adenopathies, pancreatic diseases, etc.

B. Characteristics of this Classification

1. The proposed classification as indicated by its title follows a clinical approach, taking into account its pathogenesis and considering also the etiological cause, whether it is known or not. It includes the classical pathogenic classification of jaundice into: hemolytic, hepatocellular, and obstructive; but, obviously significantly modified.

Our knowledge of jaundice-producing diseases has increased a great deal in the late years; as a result, the classic pathogenic concepts have become too schematic, and even inadequate to be used as the main criteria for classification. The unsuitability of such pathogenic concepts for a satisfactory classification is among other reasons due to: (1) The slight difference that often exists between hepatocellular and cholestatic intrahepatic jaundice and, particularly between the latter and extrahepatic jaundice; (2) the fact that some cases of hepatocellular jaundice show hemolytic signs, that is to say with indirect hyperbilirubinemia: this occurs in the diseases listed above under B.2.a.1a) and 2b) (especially caused by the inhibiting factor of the glucorinization of the mother's milk), and (3) that the icterus-producing diseases quite often exhibit all three elements of the pathological physiology of the increase of bilirubin in blood, which are indicated in the pathogeny of the icterus sign (p. 12).

We believe that, at least for the moment, in the present state of our knowledge and especially in the particular case of neonatal jaundice prolonged into infancy, the pathogenesis of icteric diseases is better classified as: by hemolysis, hepatic and by obstruction of the external ducts; subdividing the hepatic diseases into dysmetabolic, simple-inflammatory, atresia-inducing inflammatory, fibrocirrhotic, properly malformative, and intrahepatic obstructive. It must also be understood that a correlation can exist among these diseases, especially among the dismetabolic and the primarily inflammatory jaundice; thus, an incterus due to a metabolic dysfunction in galactosemia or ornitinemia can be accompanied by an inflammatory component, and jaundice due to an inflammatory process is usually accompanied by a dismetabolic component, etc.

2. We consider too schematic the most recent classification by LÜDERS [1967] into *jaundice with predominantly indirect bilirubin,* and *jaundice with predominantly direct bilirubin.* As has been pointed out by recognized authors [POPPER and SCHAFFNER, 1957] a predominance of indirect bilirubin may exist in jaundice with blood bilirubin values exceeding 3–5 mg%. In fact, in the study of 38 cases of neonatal hepatitis performed by SILVERBERG and CRAIG [1959], it was found that only half the

cases yielded a direct bilirubin/total bilirubin ratio higher than 50%. Similarly, in a recent study by SHARP et al. [1967a], in four out of ten cases there was a slight predominance of indirect bilirubin.

3. Ambiguous terms, such as pseudoobstructive or pseudomalformative jaundices do not figure in our classification. They may only be acceptable as initial, transitory terms to describe a jaundice-producing process which is being studied and awaits an accurate diagnosis which we will attempt to obtain with a minimum delay.

4. As can readily be inferred, the group of intrahepatic obstructive icterus has been drastically limited and has been reduced to a group of rare diseases[1].

A good number of authors greatly increase the range of this group, because they admit that the great majority of disease belonging to groups 2, 3b and those belonging to group 5 (omitting from the latter, extrahepatic atresia) ought to be considered pathogenically as intrahepatic obstructive, due to intrahepatic cholestasis, in contrast to classic cholestasis or extrahepatic obstruction. In our opinion, such a consideration is clearly excessive as it will be shown below.

The etiological agents of the icterus-producing diseases (congenital or, better still, *dysgenic* – by alteration of the genes – causes, and *acquired* ones: microbian, viral, chemical, etc.) act mainly in two ways from a pathogenic point of view: causing a metabolic disorder or an inflammatory injury, both of them manifested by physiological changes which lead to a hypo- or acholeresis (by acholeresis we mean the whole cycle of production and excretion of bile). Such changes certainly constitute a dysfunction or, more accurately, a combination of dysfunctions which, following a topographic-anatomical order, are: a smaller uptake of blood (indirect) bilirubin; a deficiency in the conjugation of bilirubin; difficulty

1 The marked or predominant obstruction of the bile ducts allows us to include in this group some of the cytomegalic inclusion hepatitis, such as the case recently reported by ODIÈVRE et al. [1970] where the blockage by cellular thrombi seems to be the main cause for cholestasis.

The greatly debated disease 'inspissated bile syndrome' can, in our opinion, be provisionally included in this group. Such a term should still be better defined because, as BRENT [1962] has pointed out, it constitutes a 'pigment of the imagination'. Many authors agree that with such a term one does not mean the production of an originally thick bile; the first thing would be the cholestasis – the production of the thrombi comes later [POPPER and SCHAFFNER, 1957]. It might perhaps occur so extensively that similarly to what happens in the case of obstruction by cytomegalic thrombi, it could become a fundamental pathogenic factor linked with diverse etiologies: isoimmunization, neonatal viral hepatitis, etc.

of passage through the membrane; production of a thicker bile (by diminishing the amount of water or perhaps due to the addition of a greater amount of proteins resulting from an inflammatory process or other causes), etc. Through these mechanisms, a cholestasis can result, as evidenced by the presence of bile in the liver cells or in the excretory structures. Such a static bile could undoubtedly cause obstruction (just as the exudate in the portal spaces around the bile ducts in cases of inflammation can cause or rather produce a compression) and constitutes a link in the vicious cycle which will intensify the blockage of the bile circulation and eventually the pathological process. Since such an obstruction is a secondary element in the cholestatic process, it *cannot* be considered as a fundamental pathogenic element to be used as a criterion for the classification. We believe, nevertheless, that this can be the case in some of the diseases of group 6, and even with certain restrictions for some of them, as we have seen in footnote 1.

5. According to the classic conception, extrahepatic atresia ought to be placed in group 7, as an intrinsic obstruction; intrahepatic atresia ought to be placed in the group of the intrahepatic obstructives, and neonatal hepatitis could be included in the common inflammatory jaundice. However, if we classify them in this way it leads us to believe that the three entities are independent from each other, which in our opinion is not in agreement with the observed facts.

6. We have classified in a special pathogenic group – actually a subdivision within hepatic icterus – the inflammatory and atresia-inducing triad, departing in this conception from any previous classification. Apart from the reasons to be mentioned later on to justify it, *such a group constitutes,* with the exception of the jaundice due to isoimmunization, *90% of the icterus of the newborn.* The reports by GELLIS *et al.* [1954], those of GERRISH and COLE [1951], and GROSS [1953], according to the calculations of SILVERBERG *et al.* [1960], show that extrahepatic atresia constitutes 60–65% of all cases of obstructive jaundice in the newborn [75% according to SILVERBERG *et al.,* 1960] and the remaining is distributed as follows: two thirds are due to neonatal hepatitis and one third to a miscellany: syphilis, galactosemia, etc., and intrahepatic atresia – the latter entity being much rarer than the other two, extrahepatic atresia and neonatal hepatitis.

7. It will seem a contradiction to classify in hepatic icterus the extrahepatic atresia. But as we shall see later, in the majority of cases of extrahepatic atresia there is an associated intrahepatic atresia; and even with-

out this, there are always clear signs of an inflammatory and atresia-inducing hepathopathy. Therefore, *this extrahepatic atresia constitutes an epiphe nomenon of this hepatopathy, although it is not a feature of little importance as it affects structures of such relevant anatomic and functional significance.*

8. The clinical-pathogenic-etiological classification we propose is considered more useful than the preceding ones based on the classic pathogeny of icteric diseases, or on the characteristics of a physiopathological feature, hyperbilirubinemia.

II. *Physiopathological Mechanisms of Jaundice, Main Sign in Each Entity of the Triad*

A. Bile Elaboration

It is generally accepted that the bile production cycle and its transport into the duodenum is divided into the following stages: (1) uptake by the liver cell of indirect bilirubin and cellular transport to the microsomes (lisosomes); (2) conjugation in these ultrastructural organelles; (3) intracellular transportation of conjugated bilirubin and secretion through the membrane, and (4) passage through the excreting system; from the intercellular, intervillous spaces, following the path of the canaliculli, canal of Hering, etc., until the duodenum is reached.

We give here only an outline of the bile elaboration process considering only the production of pigment, as other components of bile (water, proteins, bile salts, cholesterine, enzymes, etc.) have not been taken into account, and admitting that bilirubin glucuronization occurs inside the cell, which may not be true [COSSEL, 1965].

This process of bile production which we have described does not explain one of the unknown facts which even today exists: the presence of quite an important amount of unmodified bilirubin in the already excreted bile [COSSEL, 1965].

B. Pathogeny of Jaundice

Theoretically, icterus can be due to: (1) excessive presence of indirect bilirubin – (a) absolute, due to hemolytic increase, or (b) relative, due to reduced uptake of bilirubin or difficulty of passage through the membrane; (2) defect in conjugation at the microsome level; (3) defect in secretion-excretion = bile retention = cholestasis (a) due to a difficulty of intracellular transport of conjugated bilirubin (?); (b) due to a difficulty of passage through the membrane[2]; (c) due to a difficulty of bile circulation or transport through excretory structures at one or more of the following points – canaliculus; canal of Hering; ducts of conjunctive spaces, and great intrahepatic and extrahepatic ducts (fig. 1).

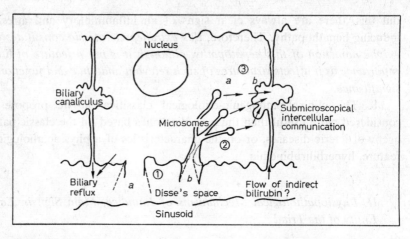

Fig. 1. Liver Cell.

Unmodified bilirubin which has not entered the cell, that which belongs to the cell, modified or not, and that which has reached the excretory ducts, passing directly or indirectly through the limphatic drainage, will produce an increase of the pigment in the blood.

The liver cell shows a *functional polarity*, with a *basal* or *sinusoidal pole* (part of the cell close to the sinusoid) and an *apical* or *biliary pole* (part of the cell surrounding the canaliculus), manifested by the cellular structure and the situation of its enzymatic system. In human cholestatic hepatosis, in hepatitis whether accompanied by cholestasis or not, and in obstructive jaundice, an inversion of the functional polarity, demonstrable both morphologically (with the electron microscope) and cytochemically is found. The polar orientation of the lysosomes in a crown around the biliary pole disappears and they appear scattered irregularly in the protoplasm. Minkowski's old theory of *paracholia* acquires then a new facet thanks to modern technical resources [Lapp, 1963].

2   These mechanisms of intracellular transport and bilirubin secretion through the membrane are so little known that Magnenat et al. [1967], who have applied the electron microscope to the study of the ultrastructural changes in cases of *chronic cellular* icterus, such as Gilbert's, Criggler-Najjar's, Dubin-Johnson's and Rotor's diseases concluded by saying that in these two last conditions there is a defect in the transport of bile from the liver cell to the canaliculus, without stating where the defect lays, whether in the intracellular transport or in the passage across the membrane. The fact that bile is not visible through the electron microscope makes it difficult to establish this point. Bile may only become visible when it joins cytoplasmic components [Hollander and Schaffner, 1968], i.e. in pathological conditions.

C. Fundamental Determinism of Jaundice in Each Entity

1. *Extrahepatic biliary atresia*, as a genuine expression of an impediment to the circulation of the bile similar to that which occurs by an obstruction, extrahepatic or intrahepatic of the corresponding ducts or by their experimental ligation.

2. *Neonatal hepatitis*, roughly considered as a hepatocellular icterus, as a disease of the liver cell proper: it is not capable of eliminating conjugated bilirubin, apart from the fact that the process of conjugation itself may be more or less deteriorated; this is supported by the high unconjugated bilirubin levels in blood which sometimes accompany this neonatal hepatitis.

3. *Intrahepatic atresia*, included in the group of icterus due to *intrahepatic cholestasis*, which SHERLOCK [1963] has qualified as 'bile secretory deficiency' and POPPER and SCHAFFNER [1957] as 'the phenomenum produced by interference in the bile flow from its formation by the liver cell', due to an anomaly in the function of the intracellular transport of conjugated bilirubin and in the secretion through the membrane and/or transport through the intrahepatic excretory ducts.

No doubt that the obliteration of the portal ducts (interlobular ducts) whose absence or great deficiency in number is the particular feature of intrahepatic atresia, will have to be considered responsible for the bile secretory deficiency of such an entity once it reaches its final stages, when all inflammatory infiltrative signs have subsided and the portal spaces only exhibit a more or less apparent fibrosis, in which period jaundice is scarcely apparent in many cases.

Nevertheless, in the progressive stage, when jaundice is much more manifest, the site of cholestasis should be located, at least in most cases, in the canaliculi or in the hepatic cells themselves, as shown by the fact that the ducts and ductules (perilobular ducts) which persist or constitute a manifestation of regeneration are almost never seen to be full of bile, and even more rarely are they found to be cystic, as would be expected if the impediment of bile circulation would lay in the atresic ducts. In fact, if some ducts or ductules have a larger diameter, they are habitually void of pigment.

To us there is no doubt that, in the ascending period of the process, when jaundice is more severe, it is produced more by the lesions of the liver cells than by the atresia of the ducts. We have good examples of intrahepatic cholestasis, in which until recently (see below) no injury of the corresponding excretory structures has been found: (1) cholestatic viral hepatitis – some authors [DUBIN *et al.*, 1960] have pointed out an increase, instead of a decrease, in the portal ductules; (2) hepatosis due to hormonal changes in pregnancy; (3) drug-induced hepatosis, especially by chlorpromazine; (4) inborn metabolic errors – galactosemia and ornithinemia, and (5) familial intrahepatic cholestasis [JUBERG *et al.*, 1966].

Finally, our assertion is supported by the observation of the 'zonal atresia' of BENAVIDES *et al.* [1962] in which the atresia appeared in a second biopsy coinciding with a clinical improvement, a paradoxical situation characterized by less ducts, with less symptomatology. COTTON's [1960] observation is similar: When there is jaundice, inflammatory cellular infiltration and many ducts are found in the portal spaces; after some years without jaundice, both the infiltration and the ducts have disappeared (disuse due to an 'absence of linkage' with the canaliculi, has brought about an atrophy, as this author says).

Furthermore, SHERLOCK [1969] has recently emphasized the frequency and the importance of the lesions which can be observed in the intrahepatic bile ducts in drug-induced, hormonal, etc., jaundice; with this it must be understood that such processes are not so strikingly different from intrahepatic atresia as it might seem at first sight.

The physiopathological elements determining icterus in each one of the entities of the triad that we have labeled as 'fundamental' must also be taken with a temporal meaning of *initial* factors. Because, as is well known, and especially demonstrable in the case of external cholestasis, a bile retention due to secondary alteration of the liver cell will occur sooner or later, as may be shown among other features by a defect in bilirubin conjugation. Using Eberlein's method, which allows the dosification of all three bilirubins (free, mono, and biconjugated), it can be proved [GERBASI, 1969] that in extrahepatic atresia, with time, the amount of monoglucuronic bilirubin increases progressively. And in the later stages when the metabolic disorder has become more marked, the levels of unmodified bilirubin can even surpass those of the modified bilirubin, especially when bilirubinemia is high, above 3–5 mg%.

The pathological process usually involves other structures, and this is especially evident in those situated above the source of injury: in injuries to external or internal excretory ducts, alterations of the liver cell will appear.

Although not quite so evident, secondary changes in the structures distal to the site of injury can also be noted, i.e. alterations of the ducts as a result of injuries to the liver cell. It is the opinion of some authors, particularly in the case of the internal ducts, that lack of use can bring about a hypoplasia, or, more accurately, a hypotrophy, according to the aphorism that 'the function creates the organ'. Nevertheless, we believe that if such ducts show lesions, they should be attributed to a pathological agent which damaged them directly.

III. Clinical Signs and Laboratory Findings

Table I shows the most outstanding sign and some of the humoral factors of each one of the entities of the triad.

Table I. Jaundice and some analytic data of the icteric inflammatory-atresying entities

	Extrahepatic atresia	Neonatal hepatitis	Intrahepatic atresia
Jaundice			
Appearance	usually within 15 days of birth[1]	usually within 15 days of birth[1]	usually within 15 days of birth[1]
Intensity	rapidly increasing	rapidly increasing	rapidly increasing
Course	almost invariably to cirrhosis	tendency to lessen and disappear in weeks or months	tendency to lessen
Laboratory findings			
Feces			
Bilirubin and stercobilin	usually not present	often present	sometimes found
Urine			
Urobilin	usually not present	often present	sometimes found
Blood			
Transaminase	late rise	rises usually early	variable
[131]I-rose bengal test	elimination below 10% in 48 h	clearly above 10% in 48 h	higher elimination than in extrahepatic atresia

1 And after 2nd to 3rd day of life.

A. Clinical Signs

1. Frequency: The figures which are given for the frequency of *extra-hepatic atresia* are quite variable: SULAMAA and VISAKORPI [1964] give the figure of one case for every 34,000 infants, CAMERON and BUNTON [1960] 1/25,000–30,000; MOORE [1953] 1/20,000 – 30,000; STOWENS [1959] 1/20,000; RICKHAM and LEE [1964] 1/13,000, and LECK [1963] 1/8,000. The quoted figures for the incidence in hospital admissions are also different: SACREZ *et al.* [1957] rates it as 0.2% and ASTRACHAN [1955] as 1.48%.

We have been unable to find any data relating to the frequency of *neonatal hepatitis*. However, bearing in mind the data of SILVERBERG *et al.* [1960], we know it is less frequent than extrahepatic atresia, the ratio being 1:2. On the other hand, DANKS [1965], in a review of 430 cases of obstructive jaundice, including his own and those of other authors, found:

	Percent
Extrahepatic atresia	47
Intrahepatic atresia	1
Neonatal hepatitis	46
Common bile duct cyst	2
Intraluminal obstruction	2
Bacterial infection	2

rating the frequency of such obstructive jaundice as 1/5,000 infants.

Intrahepatic biliary atresia as an isolated entity is quite infrequent, almost exceptional, as can be clearly seen from the findings of the authors mentioned above. PILLOUD [1966] recently compiled the great majority of recorded cases; of the 66 cases he collected, a mere 42 are classified as pure intrahepatic atresia. However, intrahepatic atresia is very frequently accompanied by extrahepatic atresia (p. 58).

2. Race and sex: The studies of BROUGH and BERNSTEIN [1969], based on confirmed cases of hepatitis and extrahepatic atresia, indicate that: (a) hepatitis affects Caucasians more frequently than negroes; the male to female ratio is higher than 2:1; (b) extrahepatic atresia affects predominantly the white race; KROVETZ [1960] already pointed this out, and although this author found no sex differences, BROUGH and BERN-STEIN [1969] pointed out a prevalence in the female sex, as did KASSAI *et al.* [1968], (c) intrahepatic atresia – ALAGILLE *et al.* [1969] found 13 boys and 12 girls among 25 cases of intrahepatic atresia.

3. The meconium, in extrahepatic atresia, according to WOLMAN [1957] can be colored green; CAMERON and BUNTON [1960] say it is usually green; KÜNZER [1962] points out that in atresia the meconium is often light grey, and that in giant cell hepatitis it is of normal color. In intrahepatic atresia, light-colored meconium has been observed by some [WILLBRANDT, 1965]. According to ALAGILLE and KREMP [1964], the meconium presents a normal aspect in atresia, although in some cases it may be abnormal; the same applies to hepatitis. Can we infer from the appearance of meconium the time of onset of the process? This is a very interesting question extensively discussed in chapter 5.III.A.1.

4. Jaundice, as shown in table I, usually appears some time after birth, i.e. these babies are not jaundiced at birth.

YLPPÖ [1913] indicated that in atresia jaundice appears most commonly between the second and fifth days of life; SILVERBERG et al. [1960] stated that it begins between the first and third week, and is often preceded by physiological jaundice; ALAGILLE and KREMP [1964] point out that in a small number of cases, jaundice is present on the first day and that in two thirds of the cases it appears within the first week. In a statistical analysis of 35 cases which included cases of atresia and others of osbtructive jaundice with a spontaneous course, GOYA et al. [1962] found that in two cases it was present at birth, in 28 it appeared together with the physiological jaundice, and in 5 it evolved 'in two stages', with a symptom-free period after the physiological icterus had disappeared. GERBASI [1969] has also stated that only in a few cases is jaundice, the main sign of biliary atresia, present at birth; in the majority of cases it appears during the first days of life.

We stated that jaundice usually appears in the period between birth (second or third day of life) and the 15th day. This constitutes grossly the average of the data supplied by various authors, and is also in agreement with our own observations. Nevertheless, in some cases jaundice has appeared at a later date; cases which show jaundice within the first 3 months are still considered as belonging to the neonatal period.

The newborn affected by one of the entities of the triad, especially in the case of extrahepatic atresia, does not frequently show jaundice at birth, for the reasons explained in chapter 6.

5. Itching: This is a symptom which can appear in all three entities, but is more frequent in intrahepatic atresia. It occurs at varying ages but generally later, in the infant period or in childhood.

Regarding its appearance in intrahepatic atresia, we can quote one of HAAS and DOABS' [1958] cases in which it appeared at five months; in another of AHRENS et al. [1951] at 1¹/₂ years, whereas in one of SHARP et al. [1967a], pruritus seems to have appeared at birth.

The variable character of this symptom and its absence in many cases of total retention (extrahepatic atresia) proves that its presence does not depend on simple cholestasis but on some of its peculiarities which are not fully understood even today. Since we have indicated that it occurs frequently in intrahepatic atresia, it may, perhaps, maintain a close relationship with a ductal-ductular hypofunction or dysfunction, as yet unknown.

For a long time, the retention of cholesterol was thought to be responsible for the itching, but it is now considered to be caused by trihydroxycholic and dihydroxycholic acids. At present [SHARP et al., 1967b], the pathophysiology of the bile acids is interpreted as follows:

The bile acids constitute one of the most important metabolic products of cholesterol. This organic alcohol produces two *primary acids,* cholic and cheno-deoxycholic, which are excreted with the bile as salts. When they reach the intestine they facilitate the absorption of fats, and are later reabsorbed in the ileum; those which are not reabsorbed are deconjugated by bacteria in the colon and transformed into *secondary bile acids,* mainly deoxycholic and lithocholic, which are also reabsorbed or eliminated with the feces. Both the primary and secondary bile acids regulate the cholesterol synthesis through a feedback mechanism. Such an enterohepatic circulation occurs approximately ten times a day.

The bile acids accumulated in the skin irritate the nerve endings and have been considered responsible for itching in liver illnesses. SCHOENFIELD et al. [1967] have proved that a close correlation exists between bile acids in the skin and pruritus. And it has also been known for a long time that the administration of unsaturated fatty acids and exchange resins (e.g. cholestyramine) are accompanied by an improvement or the disappearance of pruritus. In the 5 patients with ductipenia studied by SHARP et al. [1967a] who suffered from intense itching, a high trihydroxycholic-dihydroxycholic content was found in blood, with a trihydroxy-dihydroxy ratio higher than one. The average figures which SHARP et al. give for adults are the following:

Trihydroxy: 1.4, range 3.0–0 μg/ml
Dihydroxy: 0.76, range 2.5–0 μg/ml

According to CAREY [1958], an index higher than one in the trihydroxy-dihydroxy ratio demonstrates a hepatic illness.

Deleterious action of the secondary bile acids on the liver: The secondary bile acids constitute noxious elements for the liver.

JAVITT [1966] injected taurolithocholic acid into rats and observed a lessening in the bile flow and in the excretion of bile acids; the continuous infusion was accompanied by an increase in direct and indirect blood bilirubin and in 5-nucleotidase (an indicator enzyme). If equimolecular quantities of taurocholate and taurolithocholate are infused at the same time, such changes in the blood bilirubin do not occur. The identification of a toxic or aberrant bile acid, such as lithocholic acid, can help towards an explanation of those patients' pathology.

Apart from the experimental data, there are facts which prove lithocholic acid to be harmful to adults. In young children and infants, nevertheless, this aberrant chemical agent does *not* seem the most probable one, as this acid has not been found in infants; deoxycholic acid is only found after the first year of life. From this fact, we infer that these secondary bile acids should not be considered as the agents causing liver disorders during infancy.

Other Pathological Signs that May Occur in the
Skin following Bile Retention

Due to acid bile and cholesterol retention (and of other lipids = lipidemia increase), a dry, thickened, hardened skin with a tendency to chap, is produced. When lipidemia is very high, above 20 g/liter and it lasts for a long time, 6 months or more, it determines the production of cutaneous xanthomata; if it reaches only levels between 13 and 18 g/liter, the deposit is limited to the eyelids. No xanthomata appear if lipidemia is below 13 g/liter [AHRENS and KUNKEL, 1949].

Secondary to itching, injuries due to scratching with eventual infection are produced, habitually of the impetigo type.

6. Familial presentation: In each of the entities, familial cases have been described, especially in neonatal hepatitis. This frequency is such that for some authors [DANKS and BODIAN, 1963] it would argue in favor of a recessive hereditary factor which would manifest itself by an enzymatic defect, constituting the disease's fundamental cause which could be set off by a virus.

7. Consanguinity of the parents: In a small proportion of cases of neonatal hepatitis (4 out of 45), DANKS and BODIAN [1963] found consanguinity of the parents, a feature which according to the theory of JONES *et al.* [1968] would be peculiar to hepatitis and missing in atresia. Nevertheless, the authors do not give a statistical evaluation which could substantiate the significance of this datum.

Extrahepatic Pathological Signs
1. Nonmalformative

Each of the entities of the triad may show extrahepatic manifestations of different types: (1) digestive – vomiting, diarrhea, splenic hyperplasia, etc., and (2) neurological – especially in cases of hepatitis, but not exclusively in this entity. In intrahepatic atresia, a very characteristic clinical syndrome develops in the course of time (retarded growth, radiological skeletal changes, etc.) with peculiar facies (sunken orbits under a protruding forehead, prominent nose with a sharp ridge, slight retrognathia) which may suggest the diagnosis, before the complementary examinations permit to firmly establish it [ALAGILLE *et al.*, 1969]. In patients with an incorrectable atresia, after the age of 7 month cyanosis and clubbing of fingers and toes occurs frequently, probably due to arterial oxygen insaturation [KOBAYASHI and OHBE, 1974].

2. Malformative

Both atresia and hepatitis can be accompanied by defects in organic development, most commonly heart defects of blastoembryopathic nature[3]; certainly they are true malformations, not deformations.

The presence of a congenital anomaly, according to MYERS et al. [1956], can be suggestive in diagnosing atresia; the authors, almost without exception, have observed a high percentage of organ malformations accompanying atresia. MOORE [1953] found in his study on 31 cases of atresia, 5 cases (16%) with various anorectal, urinary and cardiac malformations. STOWENS [1959] mentions that congenital biliary atresia is accompanied in 25% of cases by malformations of other parts of the body. RUMMLER [1961] , in 18 cases of atresia, finds other malformations in 10, and in 2 out of 3 cases of familial atresia; this author considers that if a patent ductus botalli is considered as a malformation, the proportion of malformations in biliary atresia reaches the figure of 57% rather than 43%.

On the other hand, SILVERBERG et al. [1960] in a study of 38 cases of neonatal hepatitis, found 7 instances of extrahepatic malformations (18.5%).

HAYS et al. [1967] found a relative absence of other congenital anomalies, both in hepatitis and in atresia. In 71 cases of atresia they found other malformations in only 7 – a little less than 10%. Evidently, the incidence of anomalies associated with hepatitis and atresia is clearly inferior to that which the same authors find in esophagic atresia, which renders the following figures: 30% of urinary malformations; 20% of cardiac malformations; 15% of muscular skeletal ones; and 10% of the CNS. Nevertheless, the incidence of congenital malformations accompanying atresia or hepatitis indicated by HAYS et al. [1967] is still clearly higher than that given for the general population, which LUNDSTRÖM [1962] estimated at 4%.

As far as intrahepatic atresia is concerned, in PILLOUD's [1966] review of 42 cases of such an isolated atresia, he found that 10 coexisted with malformations (23.8%).

Finally, the most eloquent statistics of the presence of malformations concomitant with the entities of the triad are those of ALAGILLE et al. (1969) and ALAGILLE and KREMP [1964] found developmental anomalies in 12 cases (23%) among 52 cases of atresia, most of which corresponding

3   Regarding the blastoembryopathy related to extrahepatic atresia, the very recent contribution of LILLY and STARZL [1974] is of interest. The authors observed in a good number of cases vascular anomalies also present in normal subjects. However, the anomaly – composed of an absence of the vena cava, the preduodenal porta and anomalies of the hepatic artery affecting about 10% of the cases – has only been seen in patients with extrahepatic atresia.

to the extrahepatic type, and in 12 (13%) of 92 hepatitis cases. ALAGILLE *et al.* [1969] found 28% of cases with cardiac malformations in a series of 25 cases of intrahepatic atresia; in a good number of them other malformations, such as hypospadias, brain hypoplasia, etc. were present.

These figures indicate quite clearly that in a relevant number of cases of the three diseases of the triad, manifestations of a teratogenic action can be found. Such figures are statistically significant ($p < 0.01$). Therefore, the interrelation between accompanying malformations and entities of the triad will have to be judged according to the following possibilities:

a) *That the cause of the malformation, and that which produces the hepatopathy are different,* the latter acting on a relatively larger number of teratologically marked individuals than in healthy ones; this would mean that those affected by malformations are more susceptible to the diseases of the triad.

This hypothesis appears to be acceptable because, as is well known, many malformed individuals are especially susceptible to other morbid agents. Let us say, nevertheless, in this respect, that although among the accompanying malformations, the cardiac pathology predominates (as can be inferred from the information supplied by different authors), there is a great disparity in the various series, a heterogeneity which does not fit in with the theory that they correspond to a definite etiology[4]. For this reason in the majority of cases, the cause of such malformations cannot be suspected. Only in a very limited number of cases the entities of the triad are accompanied by a specific malformation; this is the case, for instance, of the dysontogeny due to trisomy 18.

b) *Both the malformations and the entities of the triad are due to a common cause,* which is quite obvious only in a few rare instances, as for example those of hepatitis or atresia concomitant with a typical rubella embryopathy. The lack of accompanying malformations may be due to one of the following facts: (a) The pathological stimulus appeared after the embryological period; at this stage it does not alter the morphogeny, acting only on the already formed and specially vulnerable structures. (b) The pathological stimulus does not act dysontogenetically, due to a lack of host susceptibility. In every *acquired* malformative disease (or even in nonmalformative diseases, as is already known and which is more remarkable) the susceptibility constitutes a more or less evident factor, which is probably always present. According to LANDAUER [1960] the malformation does not only depend on the moment at which the environ-

---

4   On the other hand, heart malformations are observed both in developmental disorders due to dysgenesis, e.g. mongolism, and due to acquired causes, such as rubella.

mental agent acts, but on genetic factors that direct and compensate for the harm done by it, as has been demonstrated in Drosophila; on the contrary, by the action of environmental factors, genetically preformed hereditary characters may be produced or deleted [NACHSTEIN, 1960]. WARKANY and KALTER [1961] have also pointed out the possibility of an interaction between exogenous and genetic factors; the latter determining the manifestations of the teratogenic effect.

With what has been said, we have started the etiological considerations on the malformations accompanying the triad, which are expanded in chapter 6.

3. Associated Diseases

JONES et al. [1968] drew attention to the very common association of various pathological manifestations with hepatitis, but not with atresia.

In the analysis of such diseases according to a more recent communication of DANKS [1969], one can include them in two groups: (1) constituted by diseases of proven dysgenic nature, such as mongolism, fibromatosis, cystinosis, pancreatic cystic fibrosis, etc., and (2) in which are included structural malformations not necessarily dysgenic, especially heart defects, i.e. the diseases frequently associated with atresia.

Whether the diseases of the first group constitute an etiological element of hepatitis, as JONES et al. [1968] claim, cannot be ascertained at present. For the time being, a statistical proof of these opinions is still lacking. Perhaps, the diseases associated with hepatitis will have to be properly considered as predisposing etiological factors, but not as determining or causal ones; only exceptionally in these dysgenic diseases – specifically in the two most frequent, mongolism and pancreatic cystic fibrosis – is there a concomitance with neonatal hepatitis.

B. Laboratory Data

In few areas has biochemistry been used so much and with such little result as in the diagnosis of liver diseases [WITH, 1968]. The multiple laboratory tests used to differentiate the illnesses of the parenchyma from those of the bile ducts in adults have proved, with few exceptions, to be of little value and sometimes extremely misleading in children, in particular in the field we are concerned with, of great importance and transcendency from various points of view and especially for the differential diagnosis between hepatitis and atresia. Do the modern tests introduced in the study of liver pathology, specially the exploration with radioactive iodinated rose bengal, offer better prospects for the diagnosis? Let us see some details and considerations concerning the laboratory investigations of patients affected by the triad.

1. Bilirubin and its Derivate Compounds in the Feces

With the intention of evaluating in an adequate fashion the results of the examination, the following points must be clearly understood:

a) Normally, there is always bilirubin in the feces before the end of the third month; the pigment disappears between the third and twelfth months.

b) The presence of stercobilin in the feces indicates that a reduction process of the bilirubin takes place in the intestine, to convert it into stercobilinogen, followed by an oxidative process, to transform the latter into stercobilin.

c) The conversion of bilirubin into stercobilinogen and stercobilin in the infant takes place at a slow rate; in artificially fed babies it begins towards the third day of life, and in breast-fed babies, in the second week or later.

d) The disappearance of bilirubin means that total conversion of intestinal bilirubin into stercobilinogen and stercobilin takes place.

e) Considering that urobilinogen and urobilin are nothing else than stercobilinogen and stercobilin absorbed from the gut and eliminated later on by the kidney, it may be understood, without further explanation, how the semiology of urobilinogenuria and urobilinuria should be interpreted.

1. The presence of *bile in the feces* would prove the *non total* character of jaundice, thus, extrahepatic atresia could be discarded [HSIA and GELLIS, 1953].

Let us reaffirm, however, that when talking about bile, we must refer to bilirubin, which we will have to demonstrate by more precise methods. We believe that the use of the dyazoic reactive, following the Hymans van den Berg technique is extremely reliable. On occasions, the feces are definitely colored even with a deep greenish hue, due primarily to the presence of stained mucus. This could mislead one into thinking that the ducts are patent. Such feces do *not* give a positive dyazoic reaction, neither direct nor indirect. In some of our observations, especially in two of them, one of extrahepatic atresia and another of neonatal hepatitis with marked lesions of the intrahepatic ducts, we were able to observe repeatedly the passage of feces with abundant amounts of greenish mucous material, which never gave positive bilirubin reactions. The lack of stercobilin led us to think that the color of this material had to do with oxidated bilirubin, i.e. biliverdin originated in the stained intestinal mucosa.

Such a diagnostic importance has been attributed to the presence or absence of bile in the feces that POTTS [1959] considered that one of the desirable goals of science was to find a test capable to ascertain categorically whether feces contained bile or not. We believe that it is of value to determine whether the feces contain bilirubin or not. But we cannot consider its absence as a definite proof of atresia nor its presence as a sure sign of the patency of the ducts. NORRIS and HAYS [1957] and KASSAI *et al.* [1968] pointed out a long time ago that the presence of bilirubin does not definitely rule out atresia. PILLOUD [1966b] insists on this, pointing out the deceptive character of such a fact. How, in cases of hepatitis, bilirubin can be absent from the feces is unanimously attributed to total cholestasis; and the fact that in a case of atresia – later confirmed by surgical exploration, cholangiography and liver biopsy and/or an autopsy – bilirubin can be present in feces, may have two explanations: (1) atresia was not fully defined at the moment of performing the pigment test, and (2) bilirubin is eliminated by the intestine: the indirect bilirubin by true excretion, as KÜNZER [1962] has seen in cases of hemolitic jaundice in newborn and young infants; the direct type and also the indirect one by imbibing the epithelium when this layer falls out physiologically.

2. Stercobilinogen-stercobilin determination, in the feces: Its value is limited in very small infants, due to the fact that the normal figures are low; moreover, the administration of antibiotics reduces its formation, due to the inhibition of the intestinal flora.

2. *Urine*

a) Bile pigments: The presence of bile pigments in the urine usually follows their increase in blood. Nevertheless, as the renal clearance of pigments is higher for biconjugated bilirubin, it is conceivable that when, in the course of the process, the hepatic glucuronization diminishes, even in an infant remarkably icteric, the urine pigments may become less positive and even turn negative to testing by usual reagents which react mostly to biconjugated bilirubin.

b) Urobilinogen = urobilin in urine: It can be found especially in hepatitis, but also in atresia.

HSIA and GELLIS [1953] in 26 cases of atresia find urobilinogen in the urine in 8 of them; NORRIS and HAYS [1957] find positive tests for bile in feces in 4 out of 48 cases of atresia and urobilinogen in the urine in 4 out of 27, and HAYS *et al.* [1967] indicate that the finding of urobilinogen or bilirubin in feces and of urobilinogen in the urine was made in 8 out of 14 cases of atresia. Our observations agree with these data; one of our cases with total atresia repeatedly showed an intense urobilinuria.

3. *Blood Bilirubin* (see p. 8 and 14)

As has already been mentioned, both bilirubins, direct and indirect, are involved usually with predominance of the first one. Let us point out now that according to THALER and GELLIS [1968a–d] in no case of total obstruction is the bilirubin below 4 mg%; and a complete bile retention seems to be very rare when the blood level is below this figure, although a higher one does not necessarily prove the converse. Bilirubinemia usually reaches its highest levels in atresia; nevertheless, it does not tend to surpass certain figures, between 12 and 35 mg% even when the cholestasis lasted for years [KÜNZER , 1962].

CHRISTY and BOLEY [1958] have followed 16 out of 37 cases with a proved atresia and in 6 not only was there no progressive bilirubin rise, but it decreased in a remarkable way; this by no means refers to the lowering of blood levels at the final stage, shortly before death as has been pointed out by many authors. This leads us to admit that there must be some metabolic path for the transformation of bilirubin into colorless products.

4. Bile in the Contents of a Duodenal Aspiration

In atresia, bile can be found in the aspirated duodenal contents and it may even increase after the administration of cholagogues [GELLIS and SILVERBERG]; the explanation of this fact has been discussed in the previous pages. In proved cases of hepatitis, as in the great majority of those of atresia, the feces can be pale for months and bile is often not found in the contents of the duodenal aspiration neither with nor without cholagogues.

5. Serum Enzymes in the Triad

The enzymes elaborated by the liver that can be present in the plasma are divided into 3 groups [RICHTERICH, 1965]: (1) *Secretory or incretory enzymes.* These are enzymes synthesized by the liver and poured into the bloodstream to perform their function there or at a distance, e.g. cholinesterase, ceruloplasmin and coagulation factors. These enzymes can be considered to have a function similar to that of other substances elaborated by the liver cell, such as albumin and fibrinogen. (2) *Marker or revealing enzymes.* These are enzymes elaborated by the liver cell to perform their function in the cell itself; they can pass into the plasma, but do not have any function in it. Examples of such enzymes are: GO and GP transaminases, ornithine-carbamyltransferase, leucine aminopeptidase and glutamatedehydrogenase. These enzymes can be considered to have a similar function to other substances such as vitamin B_{12}, Fe and nucleotides. These enzymes are present in very small quantities in the plasma, but can increase in a remarkable way when there is a cell injury or a simple membrane alteration of the liver cell. (3) *Excretory or eliminating enzymes.* These are enzymes which are physiologically eliminated with the bile, such as alkaline phosphatase, ceruloplasmin and leucine aminopeptidase. They can be considered as equivalent to other substances which also figure in the bile: cholesterol, bilirubin glucuronides, and urobilinogen.

Some enzymes belong to more than one category: leucine aminopeptidase corresponds to groups 2 and 3; ceruloplasmin to groups 1 and 3; alkaline phosphatase of the liver cell to groups 3 and 1.

Some enzymes are organ-specific to the liver itself, e.g. ornithine carbamyl-transferase, cholinesterase. And some are liver-specific isoenzymes, e.g. alkaline phosphatase of the excretory ducts, the so-called 'alkaline phosphatase of the cholestasis'.

a) Value of Transaminase as a Diagnostic Test

The glutamic-oxaloacetic and glutamic-pyruvic transaminases have been extensively investigated in the study of the entities of the triad in the hope that they might help to establish a differential diagnosis between them; for this reason we consider them in detail.

KOWE et al. [1958, 1960, 1963] have recommended repeated serum transaminase determinations from the onset of the icteric syndrome with the aim of distinguishing atresia from hepatitis. However, according to SILVERBERG et al. [1960] and confirmed by BENNET [1964] and SALAZAR DE SOUZA and SANCHES [1965] among others, the results obtained are so variable that their diagnostic value is very limited, especially when the jaundice has been present for some time.

The diagnostic value of the serum transaminase levels have been recently commented on by GERBASI [1969] as follows:

1. In *hepatitis*, the determination of serum transaminase levels, so useful in viral hepatitis in older children and adults, is of little or no value in the first weeks of life. This is due to the facts that: (a) high levels are not exclusive of the disease, as they can also be present in atresia, and (b) in hepatitis the high levels with inversion of the SGOT/SGPT ratio are not present, as is the case in older individuals.

2. In *atresia*, the serum transaminases constitute also an expression of liver damage, although when they increase the SGOT/SGPT ratio remains constantly above one; this ratio is maintained even in advanced phases of the process. This is why only with the presence of very high levels and a clear inversion of the rate can hepatitis be diagnosed. Nevertheless, according to GERBASI [1969], this occurs in a minority of cases.

b) Patterns of the Serum Enzyme Changes in the Entities of the Triad

RICHTERICH [1965] has worked out a table of the behavior of liver enzymes in the different clinical syndromes; table II is an abbreviated form, as published by COLOMBO [1968] and somewhat modified by us:

Table II includes one of the new excretory enzymes, γ-glutamyl transpeptidase, which recently has been introduced in the enzymatic diagnosis. This enzyme has turned out to be one of the most sensitive to disorders of drainage in the bile ducts. Its sensitivity, according to LUKASIK et al. [1968], is 6 times greater than that of alkaline phosphatase and 9 times that of leucine aminopeptidase.

Table II

Serum activity	Enzymes	Syndrome		
		a	b	c
Marker or revealing				
Increased	glutamic-oxaloacetic transaminase	+++	+	+
	glutamic-pyruvic transaminase	+++	0	0
	leucine aminopeptidase	++	++	+++
	ornithine carbamyltransferase	+++	++	++
	glutamate dehydrogenase	+	0	++
Excretory				
Increased	alkaline phosphatase	0	0	+++
	ceruloplasmin	0	0	+++
	γ-glutamyl transpeptidase	+	+	+++
Secretory (incretory)				
Decreased	cholinesterase	0	+++	0

a = Diffuse acute injury of the membrane, acute hepatitis type; b = diffuse chronic injury of the parenchyma, compensated cirrhosis type; c = obstruction of the bile ducts, extrahepatic occlusion type.

The enzymatic spectrum which results from blockage of the bile ducts becomes complex and misleading when a membrane injury due to a parenchymal alteration is added to the cholestatic process. And, conversely, a good number of cases of hepatitis or other icteric processes of the newborn or small infants frequently show a cholostatic component; for this reason, *we cannot entrust the diagnosis of atresia exclusively to the enzymatic determinations* [COLOMBO, 1968].

Recently, it has been reported that one of the alkaline phosphatase isoenzymes corresponds to the so-called 'phosphatase of the cholostasis', i.e. an alkaline phosphatase elaborated by the cells of the excretory system, cytochemically demonstrable in them and not in the hepatocyte, and usually not present in the blood. In cases of obstruction of the bile ducts significant levels of this isoenzyme may be demonstrated in blood.

Will the determination of this 'phosphatase of the cholostasis' be of value in the differential diagnosis between hepatitis and atresia? Only further experience will provide the answer to this question though, in our opinion, it will probably not be as conclusive as it might be hoped.

So far, our observations suggest that the blood rise of the isoenzyme of alkaline phosphatase elaborated by the biliary ducts may only happen in atresic cholostasis without intrahepatic atresia, accompanied by evident proliferation of biliary ductules and ducts. In two cases, the phosphatase of cholestasis was investigated: One was a case of intrahepatic biliary atresia[5] (perhaps with simultaneous extra-intrahepatic atresia as suggested by the cholangiographic image), that showed total cholostasis (2.3% ^{131}I-rose bengal eliminated through the feces in 72 h). The second was a case of hepatitis with such extensive degenerative changes in the biliary channels that they were first suggestive of evolution into extrahepatic atresia and later into intrahepatic atresia (case 16, p. 229), and practically total cholestasis (10.6% of eliminated radioiodinated rose bengal in 48 h); no phosphatase isoenzyme was demonstrated in blood in either case.

6. *Other Laboratory Data*

a) Blood chemistry, such as total proteins, colloidal lability tests (Weltmann, Takata, cadmium, thymol, cephalin, cholesterol, etc.) have proved of little value as indicators of a definite icterus-producing process and are of no use to differentiate hepatitis from atresia. Certainly, of more value, although not as a constant or exclusive feature, are the increased levels of blood lipids, especially cholesterol, which can be observed in intrahepatic atresia, especially in cases of protracted course, and also the trihydroxy and dihydroxy acids which have already been mentioned (p. 18)[6].

b) Blood cytology: No significant information can be drawn from the red or white blood cells counts. It should be pointed out that ALAGILLE *et al.* [1969] found a remarkable thrombocytosis in a good proportion of cases of intrahepatic atresia (7 out of 25). In our own observations of isolated intrahepatic atresia, we failed to find any cases of thrombocytosis, but we have found an elevated platelet count in two cases of extrahepatic atresia, one with severe deterioration of the intrahepatic ducts (case 13, p. 226) and the other with less intense ductal lesions (case 6, p. 219): a case of complete triad, where the microscopic pathology of the liver showed features of all three entities.

---

5   Not included in the case reports of this book.
6   Recently, in cases of atresia, an abnormal low density serum lipoprotein has been demonstrated: lipoprotein X. Nevertheless, it has also been demonstrated in cases of hepatitis [RAINER POLEY *et al.*, 1972]. The determination of serum levels of 5'-nucleotidase [YEUNG, 1972] that of α-fetoprotein [ZELTZER *et al.*, 1974] and certain features of hemolysis [as demonstrated by the peroxide test, LUBIN *et al.*, 1971; MELHORN *et al.*, 1972] cannot yet be considered as very accurate for such a differential diagnosis on account of the small number of studied cases.

7. Laboratory Tests Requiring Administration of Substances

a) Bromosulfophthalein test (BSP): This test is of no value.

b) Radioactive ^{131}I-rose bengal test: This test, introduced a few years ago, has proved valuable in the differential diagnosis between hepatitis and atresia [GEPPERT and BRENT, 1957; SHNUG, 1958; WHITE et al., 1963]. According to THALER and GELLIS [1968a–d] and COLOMBO [1968] it constitutes *the best diagnostic laboratory test*. Nevertheless, it is not infallible, as GHADIMI and SASS-KORTSAK pointed out soon after it was introduced; this was recently confirmed by THALER and GELLIS [1968a–d], who found that in 20% of the cases of hepatitis, the figures of elimination overlap with those of total biliary obstruction.

The evaluation of the test is centered especially on intestinal elimination: on the amount of radioactive material present in the feces during the 48 or 72 h which follow the intravenous administration of the product. SHARP et al. [1967b], in a study of the test in a good number of icterus-producing disease, found a maximal elimination of 6.5% after 48 h in 8 cases of extrahepatic atresia; THALER and GELLIS [1968a–d] quote for this type of atresia a figure below 10%, the same as DESBUQUOIS et al. [1968] (for 72 h). In the case of neonatal hepatitis the elimination figures are usually much higher, although as we mentioned exceptions are not infrequent. As for intrahepatic atresia, the elimination figures are of intermediate values, between 15 and 30% for 72 h [according to DESBUQUOIS et al., 1968].

The accuracy of the test seems to be greater if the hepatic scintography is carried out at 72 and 96 h after injection [KIMURA, 1974]. In the case of atresia the image of the liver and kidneys can be clearly observed, while in hepatitis the hepatic shadow cannot be identified in the scintigram.

Apart from the indicated efficiency, the ^{131}I-rose bengal test offers a considerable advantage: As the isotope dose that is administered is small, undesirable side effects are unlikely and the test can be repeated if necessary. These are important features of this test for the differential diagnosis.

c) Labeled cholic acid test: As an aid for the differential diagnosis between hepatitis and atresia, NORMAN et al. [1969] have tried the 24 ^{14}C-cholic acid test. The results obtained indicate that the metabolism and excretion of this acid in cases of atresia have shown similar characteristics to cases of intrahepatic cholestasis (neonatal hepatitis).

d) The vitamin E absorption test of MELHORN et al. [1972]: The reliability of this test is still to be demonstrated (only few analyzed cases up to now).

References

AHRENS, E. H., jr. and KUNKEL, H. G.: Relationship between serum lipids and skin xantomata in 18 patients with primary biliary cirrhosis. J. clin. Invest. 28: 1565 (1949).

AHRENS, E. H., jr.; HARRIS, R. C., and MACMAHOW, H. E.: Atresia of the intrahepatic bile ducts. Pediatrics, Springfield 8: 628 (1951).

ALAGILLE, D.; HABIB, E. C. et THOMASIN, N.: L'atrésie des voies biliares intrahépatiques avec voies biliaires extrahépatiques perméables chez l'enfant. A propos de 25 observations. J. Paris. Pédiat. 301 (1969).

ALAGILLE, D. et KREMP, L.: Les ictères du nouveau-né en dehors de l'incompatibilité foeto-maternelle. Données statistique. Revue int. Hépat. 14: 6 (1964).

ASTRACHAN: cit. BRUSA, P. e PARENZAN, L.: Sull'oclusione congenita delle vie billiari. Minerva paediat. 7: 851 (1955).

BENAVIDES, L.; KUMATE, J., and SALAS, M.: Zonal atresia of intrahepatic bile ducts. 10th Int. Congr. Pediatrics, Lisboa 1962, abstracts of papers, p. 244.

BENNET, D. E.: Problems in neonatal obstructive jaundice. Pediatrics, Springfield 33: 735 (1964).

BRENT, R. L.: Persistent jaundice in infancy. J. Pediat. 61: 111 (1962).

BROUGH, A. and BERNSTEIN, J.: Liver biopsy in the diagnosis of infantile obstructive jaundice. Pediatrics, Springfield 43: 519 (1969).

CAMERON, R. and BUNTON, G. L.: Congenital biliary atresia. Br. med. J. ii: 1253 (1960).

CAREY, J. B., jr.: Serum trihydroxy-dihydroxy bile-acid ratio in liver and biliary disease. J. clin. Invest. 37: 1494 (1958).

CHRISTY, R. A. and BOLEY, J. O.: The relation of hepatic fibrosis to concentration of bilirubin in the serum of congenital atresia of the biliary tract. Pediatrics, Springfield 21: 226 (1958); cit. SILVERBERG, CRAIG and GELLIS, and THALER and GELLIS.

COLOMBO, J. P.: Le diagnostique enzymatique en pédiatrie. Etude des enzymes du plasma et des cellules sanguines. Ann. Nestlé 32: 27 (1968).

COSSEL, L.: Elektromikroskopische Befunde an der Leber zur Pathogenese des Ikterus. Münch. med. Wschr. 107: 1376 (1965).

COTTON, D. A.: Intrahepatic biliary atresia. Lancet ii: 294 (1960).

DANKS, D. M.: Prolonged neonatal obstructive jaundice. A survey of modern concepts. Clin. Pediat. 4: 499 (1965).

DANKS, D. M.: Personal commun. (1969).

DANKS, D. M. and BODIAN, P. M.: A genetic study of neonatal obstructive jaundice. Archs Dis. Childh. 38: 378 (1963).

DESBUQUOIS, B.; TRON, P. et ALAGILLE, D.: Etude de l'excretion fécale et urinaire du rose de bengale marqué par l'iode radiactif au cours des ictères obstructifs du nouveau-né et du nourrison. Archs fr. pédiat. 25: 379 (1968).

DUBIN, I. N.; SULLIVAN, B. H.; LEGOLVAN, P. C., and MURPHY, L. C.: The cholestatic form of viral hepatitis. Am. J. Med. 29: 55 (1960).

GELLIS, S. S.; CRAIG, J. M., and HSIA, D. Y.: Prolonged obstructive jaundice in infancy. IV. Neonatal hepatitis. Am. J. Dis. Child. 88: 285 (1954).

GELLIS, S. S. and SILVERBERG, M.: cit. SILVERBERG, CRAIG and GELLIS.

GEPPERT, L. J. and BRENT, R. L.: Radioactive rose bengal. An aid in the differential diagnosis of the jaundiced infant. Am. J. Dis. Child. 94: 544 (1957).

GERBASI, M.: Contributo del pediatra a la diagnosi di malattie chirurgiche del fegato e delle vie biliari. Riv. Chir. pediat. 11: 224 (1969).

GERRISH, E. W. and COLE, J. W.: Surgical jaundice in infants and children. Archs Surg., Chicago 63: 529 (1951).

GHADIMI, H. and SASS-KORTSAK, A.: Evaluation of radioactive rose bengal test for the differential diagnosis of obstructive jaundice in infancy. New Engl. J. Med. 265: 351 (1961).

GOYA, N., et al.: Jap. U. Clin. exp. Med. 39: 856 (1962); cit. GERBASI.

GROSS, R. E.: The surgery of infancy and childhood, Spanish ed., p. 513 (Saunders, Philadelphia 1953).

HAAS, L. and DOABS, R.: Congenital absence of intrahepatic bile ducts. Archs Dis. Childh. 33: 396 (1958).

HAYS, D. M.; WOOLLEY, M. M.; SNYDER, W. H., jr.; REED, G. B.; GWINN, J. L., and LANDING, B. A.: Diagnosis of biliary atresia. Relative accuracy of percutaneous liver biopsy, open liver biopsy and operative cholangiography. J. Pediat. 71: 598 (1967).

HOLLANDER, M. and SHAFFNER, F.: Electron microscopic studies in biliary atresia. Am. J. Dis. Child. 116: 49 (1968).

HSIA, D. Y. and GELLIS, S. A.: Prolonged obstructive jaundice in infancy. IV. Neonatal hepatitis. Am. J. Dis. Child. 85: 13 (1953).

JAVITT, N. B.: Cholestasis in rats induced by taurolithocholate. Nature, Lond. 210: 1962 (1966).

JONES, P. G.; DANKS, D. M.; CLARKE, A. M., and CAMPBELL, P. E.: Atresia of the extrahepatic bild ducts. A study of cases proven by operative and/or autopsy, with speculation on the etiology. 12th Int. Congr. Pediat., Mexico 1968, vol. 3, p. 665.

JUBERG, R. C.; HOLLAND-MORITZ, R. M.; HENLEY, K. S., and GONZALEZ, C. F.: Familial intrahepatic cholestasis with mental growth and retardation. Pediatrics, Springfield 38: 819 (1966).

KASSAI, M.; KIMURA, S.; ASAKURA, Y.; SUKUZI, A.; TAIRA, Y., and OHASHI, E.: Surgical treatment of biliary atresia. J. pediat. Surg. 3: 665 (1968).

KIMURA, S.: The early diagnosis of biliary atresia. Acquisitions en chirurgie infantile, tome 6, p. 91 (Masson et Cie, Paris 1974).

KOBAYASHI, A. and OHBE, Y.: Cyanosis and clubbing of the fingers and toes in congenital biliary atresia. Helv. paediat. Acta 27: 203 (1972).

KOWE S.; GOLDSTEIN, S., and WROBLEWSKY, F.: Serum transaminase activity in the neonatal period. J. Am. med. Ass. 168: 860 (1958).

KOWE, S.; DISCHE, R. M., and WROBLEWSKY, F.: Early diagnosis of biliary tract malformation in newborn by serum transaminase pattern. N.Y. St. J. Med. 63: 3497 (1963).

KOWE, S.; PERRY, R., and WROBLEWSKY, F.: Diagnosis of neonatal jaundice by patterns of serum transaminase. Am. J. Dis. Child. 100: 47 (1960).

KROVETZ, L. H.: Congenital biliary atresia. II. Analysis of the therapeutic problem. Surgery, St Louis 47: 468 (1960).

KÜNZER, W.: Der Ikterus des Neugeborenen. Ein Überblick. Annls paediat. *198:* I, p. 240; II, p. 314; III, p. 375 (1962).

LANDAUER, W.: Wechselspiel zwischen genetischen und exogenen Faktoren bei der Entstehung kongenitaler Missbildungen. 1. Int. Konf. über kongenitale Missbildungen, London 1960. Schweiz. med. Wschr. *90:* 1926 (1960).

LAPP, H.: Die submikroskopische Organisation der Leberzelle. Münch. med. Wschr. *105:* 1 (1963).

LECK, .: in COUREVITCH The surgery of jaundice in the newborn, with special reference to congenital atresia of the bile ducts. Ann. R. Coll. Surg. *32:* 334 (1963).

LILLY, J. R. and STARZL, T. E.: Liver transplantation in children with biliary atresia and vascular anomalies. J. pediat. Surg. *9:* 707 (1974).

LUBIN, B. H.; BAEHNER, R. L.; SCHWARTZ, E.. SHOET, S. A., and NATAN, D. G.: The red cell peroxide hemolysis test in the differential diagnosis of obstructive jaundice in the newborn period. Pediatrics, Springfield *48:* 565 (1971).

LÜDERS, D.: Practica pediatrica; Spanish ed., p. 187 (1967).

LUKASIK, S.; RICHTERICH, R. und COLOMBO, J. P.: Der diagnostische Wert der alkalischen Phosphatase, der Leucinaminopeptidase und der γ-glutamiltranspeptidase bei Erkrankungen der Gallenwege. Schweiz. med. Wschr. *98:* 81 (1968).

LUM, C. H.; MARSHALL, W. J.; KOZAL, D. D., and MYER, K. A.: The use of radioactive (131I-labelled) rose bengal in the study of human liver diseases. Ann. Surg. *149:* 353 (1959).

LUNDSTRÖM, R.: Rubella during pregnancy. Follow-up study of children born after epidemic of rubella in Sweden 1951. With additional investigation of prophilaxis and treatment of maternal rubella. Acta paediat. scand. *51:* suppl. 133 (1962).

MAGNENAT, P.; MINIO, F. et GAUTIER, A.: Remarques sur les mécanismes des ictères hépatiques chroniques. Bull. Mém. Soc. Hôp. Paris *118:* 65 (1967).

MELHORN, K. D.; GROSS, S., and IZANT, R. J.: The red cell hydrogen peroxide hemolysis test and vitamin E absorption in the differential diagnosis of jaundice in infancy. J. Pediat. *81:* 1082 (1972).

MOORE, T. C.: Congenital atresia of the extrahepatic bile ducts. Report of 31 proven cases. Surgery Gynec. Obstet. *96:* 215 (1953).

MYERS, R. L.; BAGGENSTOSS, A. H.; LOGAN, G. B., and HALLEN BECK, G. A.: Congenital atresias of the extrahepatic biliary tract. A clinical and pathological study. Pediatrics, Springfield *13:* 767 (1956).

NACHSTEIN, H.: Wechselwirkung zwischen Gen und Milieu. 1. Int. Konf. über kongenitale Missbildungen, London 1960. Schweiz. med. Wschr. *90:* 1926 (1960).

NORMAN, A.; STRANDVIK, B., and ZETTERSTRÖM, R.: Bile acid excretion and malabsorption in intrahepatic cholestasis of infancy (neonatal hepatitis). Acta paediat., scand. *58:* 59 (1969).

NORRIS, W. and HAYS, D. M.: Problems in diagnosis associated with obstructive neonatal jaundice. Am. J. Surg. *94:* 321 (1957).

ODIÈVRE, M.; GAUTIER, M.; NORTON, F. et ALAGILLE, D.: Cholestase intrahépatique par obstruction des voies biliaires intralobulaires au cours d'une maladie généralisée des inclusions cytomégaliques chez un nouveau-né. Archs fr. Pédiat. *27:* 211 (1970).

PILLOUD, P.: Un cas de syndrome de MacMahon-Thannhauser congénitale; modalité pathogénique particulière de l'agénésie biliaire intrahépatique. Helv. paediat. Acta *21:* 327 (1966).

PILLOUD, P.: L'hépatite néo-natale. Méd. Hyg. *24:* 230 (1966b).

POPPER, H., and SHAFFNER, F.: Liver structure and function (McGraw Hill, New York 1957).

POTTS, W.: The surgeon and the child, Spanish ed., p. 168 (Saunders, Philadelphia 1959).

RAINER POLEY, J.; IDE SMITH, E.; BOON, O. J.; BHATIAS, M.; SMITH, C. W., and THOMPSON, J. B.: Lipoprotein-X and the double ^{131}I-rose bengal test in the diagnosis of prolonged infantile jaundice. J. pediat. Surg. *7:* 660 (1972).

RICKHAM, P. P. and LEE, E. Y. G.: Neonatal jaundice. Surgical aspects. Clin. Pediat. *3:* 197 (1964).

RICHTERICH, R.: Enzymdiagnostik der Leberkrankheiten. Pädiat. FortbildK. Praxis, vol. 15, p. 17 (Karger, Basel 1965).

RICHTERICH, R.: cit. COLOMBO.

RUMLER, W.: Über die kongenitale Gallengangsatresie, zum familiären Vorkommen und zur Genese dieser Fehlbildung. Arch. Kinderheilk. *161:* 238 (1961).

SACREZ, R.; FRUHLING, L. et VOGEL, R.: Les malformations des voies biliaires extrahépatiques. Pédiatrie *11:* 303 (1956).

SALAZAR DE SOUZA, J. et SANCHES, N.: Les ictères obstructifs néonataux. Pédiatrie *20:* 383 (1965).

SHARP, L. H.; CAREY, J. B.; WHITE, J. C., and KRIVIT, K.: Cholestiramine therapy in patients with a paucity of intrahepatic bile ducts. J. Pediat. *71:* 723 (1967b).

SHARP, L. H.; KRIVIT, W., and LOWMAN, J. T.: The diagnosis of complete extrahepatic obstruction by rose bengal I-131. J. Pediat. *70:* 46 (1967a).

SHERLOCK, S.: Diseases of the liver and biliary system; 2nd Spanish ed. (Blackwell, Oxford 1963).

SHERLOCK, S.: Chronic intrahepatic obstructive jaundice. Illustrated therapeutic notes. Park Davis Publ. No. 3, p. 14 (1969).

SHNUG, G. E.: Importance of early operation in congenital atresia of extrahepatic bile ducts. Ann. Surg. *148:* 931 (1958).

SHOENFIELD, L. J.; SJOVALL, J., and PERMAN, F.: Bile acids on the skin of patients with pruritic hepatobiliary diseases. Nature, Lond. *213:* 931 (1967).

SILVERBERG, M. and CRAIG, J.: cit. SILVERBERG, CRAIG and GELLIS.

SILVERBERG, M.; CRAIG, J., and GELLIS, S. A.: Problems in the diagnosis of biliary atresia. A review and consideration of histological criteria. Am. J. Dis. Child. *99:* 575 (1960).

STOWENS, D.: Diseases of the liver; in Pediatric pathology, 1st ed., p. 484 ff. (Williams & Wilkins, Baltimore 1959).

SULAMAA, M. and VISAKORPI, J. K.: Surgery of the biliary tract in early childhood. Annls Paediat. Fenn. *10:* 1 (1964).

THALER, M. M. and GELLIS, S. A.: Studies in neonatal hepatitis and biliary atresia. I. Long-term of neonatal hepatitis. Am. J. Dis. Child. *116:* 257 (1968a).

THALER, M. M. and GELLIS, S. A.: Studies in neonatal hepatitis and biliary atresia. II. The effect of diagnostic laparotomy on long-term prognosis of neonatal hepatitis. Am. J. Dis. Child. *116:* 262 (1968b).

THALER, M. M. and GELLIS, S. A.: Studies in neonatal hepatitis and biliary atresia.

III. Progression and regression of cirrhosis in biliary atresia. Am. J. Dis. Child. *116:* 271 (1968c).

THALER, M. M. and GELLIS, S. A.: Studies in neonatal hepatitis and biliary atresia. IV. Diagnosis. Am. J. Dis. Child. *116:* 280 (1968d).

WARKANY, J. and KALTER, H.: Congenital malformations. New Engl. J. Med. *265:* 993 (1961).

WHITE, W. E.; WELCH, J. S.; DARROW, D. C., and HOLDER, T. M.: Pediatric application of radioiodine (^{131}I) rose bengal in hepatic and biliary system disease. Pediatrics, Springfield *32:* 239 (1963).

WILBRANDT, W. CH.: Atresie der intrahepatischen Gallenwege in zwei Familien. Med. Klin. *60:* 409 (1965).

WITH, T. K.: Bile pigments: chemical, biological and clinical aspects, pp. 178, 669 (Academic Press, New York 1968).

WOLMAN, I. J.: Laboratory applications in clinical pediatrics, p. 494 (McGraw Hill, New York 1957).

YEUNG, C. Y.: Serum 5'-nucleotidase in neonatal hepatitis and biliary atresia. Preliminary observations. Pediatrics, Springfield *50:* 812 (1972).

YLPPÖ, A.: Zwei Fälle von congenitalem Gallengangsverschluss: Fett und Bilirubinstoffwechselversuche bei einem derselben. Z. Kinderheilk. *9:* 319 (1913).

ZELTZER, P. M.; FONKALSRUD, E. W.; NEERHOUT, R. C., et al.: Differentiation between neonatal hepatitis and biliary atresia by measuring serum alpha-fetoprotein. Lancet *i:* 373 (1974).

Chapter 2

Diagnosis of the Triad and its Entities

I. Diagnosis of the Triad's Syndrome

The diagnosis of the triad's syndrome is established on the basis of the clinical-pathogenic-etiological list. We will not attempt to discuss a differential diagnosis based only on the routine clinical and laboratory data, as these do not provide a sure diagnosis.

The diagnosis of the triad's syndrome may be established by three successive steps:

1. A probability diagnosis is reached, by excluding other icteric processes, especially the most common ones.

Physiological jaundice: As an average it lasts one week; in premature babies it lasts longer. Although the jaundice of the triad may be related to physiological jaundice it lasts much longer.

Hemolytic jaundices: The clinical picture of a jaundice of very early onset and a few pertinent laboratory data easily rule out the most common one: jaundice due to isoimmunization.

Metabolic jaundices: Ordinarily they display *jaundice of little intensity and are relatively infrequent*. The most common are secondary to other processes, particularly some congenital diseases.

Among these metabolic jaundices (not included in the clinical-pathogenic-etiological list) SUMMERSKILL and WALSHE's [1959] 'cholostatic recurrent jaundice' should be included provisionally, as up to the moment, a clearly defined pathological picture either at the optic or the electron microscope has not been described [SUMMERSKILL, 1965]. This disease, characterized by icteric 'bouts' of variable duration separated by symptom-free intervals, usually appears after sometime, although it may be already present at birth. We do not consider Byler's disease, 'familial intrahepatic cholestasis', in this differential diagnosis because here there is a late onset of jaundice towards the second third of the first year; itching may appear earlier, from the third to fifth month[7]. Nevertheless, there is a malignant form of these diseases, of earlier presentation [observations of GRAY and SAUNDERS, 1966], which certainly should be included (see definitive diagnosis of intrahepatic atresia, p. 101).

Infectious jaundices: The 'extrahepatic' symptomatology associated to the icteric process facilitates the diagnosis of the etiological agents: skin rash in the infection by the herpes virus; lesions in various body areas, in the bacterial septic jaundice; etc. Moreover, the laboratory usually identifies the etiological agent: e.g. in the case of cytomegalovirus infection, in which the characteristic inclusion bodies may be found in the urinary sediment. Let us state that the cytomegalovirus is an etiological agent of neonatal hepatitis, of 'neonatal hepatitis' itself, with transformation into giant cells; but it is doubtful that it may cause the atresying disease (chap. 7, p. 187).

The differentiation of the triad from the diseases of group 7 does not usually offer any serious difficulties. The physical examination and radiological exploration provide valuable information to reach a diagnosis; e.g. this is the case in common bile duct cyst (or pseudocyst), with the presence of an abdominal mass, intermittent jaundice, and the shape and situation (directed downwards and frontwards) of the duodenal loop, demonstrated by an upper GI series; in the case of an obstruction of the common bile duct by an annular pancreas, the double bullous image due to an associated concomitant duodenal stenosis, etc.

Differentiating the triad from the very rare diseases of groups 4, 5 and 6 is very difficult; this applies especially to the distinction between the atresia of the inflammatory and atresia-inducing disease and atresia due to dysgenesis, which is only made with certainty when the ductal atresia is accompanied by malformations of the parenchyma, and if this occurs it would be extremely unusual.

2. Special tests, like the ^{131}I-rose bengal or the needle biopsy of the liver, can lead to a *diagnosis of great probability.*

3. A correct, sure, diagnosis is obtained by surgical exploration and the study of a surgical biopsy. If the ducts fail to 'unblock' after a reasonably long time, a surgical exploration is in order with the very likely outcome of finding an atresia or perhaps an obstructive lesion of the large

7   A curious fact is that in some of these cases indistinct interlobar ducts with an almost invisible lumen and irregular, flattened epithelium have been described, i.e. with a certain ductipenia [HAYS *et al.*, 1967, chap. 1].

ducts, either extrinsic or intrinsic, not diagnosed prior to the surgical exploration and which may be amenable to surgical treatment.

The exploration of the bile ducts, the operative cholangiogram and the study of the 'surgical' liver biopsy which yields more specimen material than a percutaneous needle biopsy, will allow the confirmation of an inflammatory process with a more or less severe and extensive damage to the excretory structures. In practically all cases, a very probable or almost a sure diagnosis of entity can be reached with a surgical intervention.

In the next section we elaborate this point further.

II. Diagnosis of Each Entity of the Triad

The clinical and analytic picture is not sufficient to reach a correct diagnosis of each of the entities of the triad. Even the demonstration of bilirubin in the feces will not definitely rule out atresia; neither is the new exploratory test with ^{131}I-rose bengal free of inaccuracy; a fecal elimination of less than 10% in 48 h does not constitute an unquestionable figure of atresia. Finally, the liver needle biopsy does not constitute a decisive diagnostic element due, besides other contingencies, to the small size of the sample obtained.

A new diagnostic method, the ultrasonic echo, recently introduced by the Japanese authors SURUGA et al. [1969] (see also p. 206), seems to be capable of achieving the diagnosis of one of the entities of the triad, extrahepatic atresia being at the same time an indicator of the therapeutic possibilities prior to laparotomy.

Thus, to reach an unquestionable diagnosis or at least a very probable one, it is necessary in many cases to resort to other methods of exploration, i.e. direct inspection of the external bile ducts, cholangiography[8], and surgical biopsy.

The hazards of surgical exploration in patients with neonatal hepatitis are well known at present. We emphasize that we do not refer to the immediate complications which, thanks to progress in technique, have been practically overcome (among us, for example, GUBERN-SALISACHS [1970] has carried out more than 40 interventions in cases of protracted neonatal icteric syndromes without undesirable pre- or postoperative

8   Operative cholangiography; rarely does nonoperative cholangiography, be it by oral or intravenous route, give valuable results.

complications); we refer specifically to the possibility of producing a hepatic miopragia which may become irreversible, leading to a chronic hepatopathy with a final cirrhotic course in a good number of cases.

NORRIS and HAYS [19577, chap. 1] observed that 6 out of 8 cases of giant cell hepatitis which were laparatomized followed a chronic course ending in cirrhosis, whereas only 2 out of 13 cases not operated showed this complication. Also, the recent statistically significant data supplied by THALER and GELLIS [1968a–d, chap. 1] have clearly underlined the dangers inherent to a surgical intervention, particularly in cases of neonatal hepatitis.

According to these authors, and bearing in mind that the intervention is not innocuous, the generally favorable course of the hepatitis in the lapse of 1–3 months and that a cirrhosis resulting from atresia will not strongly deteriorate during this period of time, a surgical exploration should not be hastily undertaken. We recommend it only after $2^1/_2$–3 months if the bile ducts remain 'blocked', without any sign of recovering their patency (chap. 11).

Before resorting to surgical exploration, it may be advisable to perform a laparoscopy with laparoscopic cholangiography as recommended by LLANIO and JORDAN [1965]. The advantages of this technique are that it may be carried out under light sedation with barbiturates and chlorpromazine, without having to resort to a general anesthetic; it affords a good view of the liver with only a small incision; it allows a selective needle biopsy and a laparoscopic cholangiography may be done if indicated. The procedure can be repeated if necessary. In 40 cases studied by these authors, the results were conclusive; only in 4 were the findings dubious and it was necessary to resort to laparotomy.

Keeping these facts in mind, let us consider now the information that may be obtained by an exploratory laparotomy.

A. Direct Inspection of the Bile Ducts
By direct inspection of the external biliary tree it may be established whether or not the gallbladder and ducts have a normal aspect, and especially whether they show any signs of intrinsic or extrinsic obstruction or are more or less atresic. The conditions in which such an inspection is carried out are not favorable enough to be of absolute value.

SILVERBERG et al. [1960, chap. 1] commented that: 'The surgeon, by means of direct exploration, is apparently in the best situation to determine whether there exists any malformation of the extrahepatic biliary tree. Nevertheless, he is often uneasy because of a small and complicated operative space which can contain a small but patent ductal system or because of an operable malformation which he has to determine with precision. The majority of surgeons who have treated a good number of cases of biliary atresia have found the patient with narrow bile ducts or without bile ducts, whose icterus later disappears or in whom, in a later operation, or with cholangiography, a functioning ductal system is found.'

From this, two postulates that a surgeon must take into careful consideration can be inferred: (1) damage to the ducts in the course of the exploration must be avoided by gentle handling of the structures, and (2) the external bile ducts in the region of the hepatic and common bile ducts should never be biopsied.

B. Verification of the Patency of the Ducts by Means of Cholangiography

Various methods of cholangiography have been used by surgeons for years. When an adequate gallbladder is found, contrast material may be injected into it. Some authors have tried injecting the material via the duodenal ending of the common bile duct. The results of these techniques have been poor.

The most suitable procedure, universally accepted today, was described by SWENSON and FISHER [1955], with some modifications suggested by HARRIS et al. [1958]. These authors suggested also the practice of postoperative cholangiography. When the contrast material passes easily and freely from the gallbladder to the duodenum, but does not fill the hepatic ducts, a catheter is left in the gallbladder and contrast material is injected into it several times in the course of a week. They recommend such a course of action as in one of their cases the ducts were not demonstrated in the first cholangiography, but only in the second one. Nevertheless, SWENSON [1960] has pointed out that if the lower bile duct is clamped with a soft vascular clamp it helps in demonstrating the presence of the ducts, if they exist. Cholangiography shows not only the presence of patent ducts but may suggest the type of reconstructive procedures more likely to succeed.

With cholangiography, a valuable and trustworthy image of the external ducts may usually be obtained. Nevertheless, good results are not always obtained, either due to a technical defect or, more frequently, because the contrast material fails to fill the passages if some product of secretion, excretion or exudation fills them; therefore, operative cholangiography is not infallible.

A recent and excellent contribution to the interpretation of the images obtained by cholangiography in hepatitis or atresia is due to HAYS et al. [1967, chap. 1]. They group them into the following types:

In type A [fig. 2, copied from HAYS et al., 1967, chap. 1], a cystic structure is found which apparently corresponds to a rudimentary gallbladder accompanied in some cases by traces of hepatic or common bile ducts; such a cystic formation offers sometimes unusual forms (fig. 2, 2–4). An additional cystic formation (fig. 2, 1) can be found in the subhe-

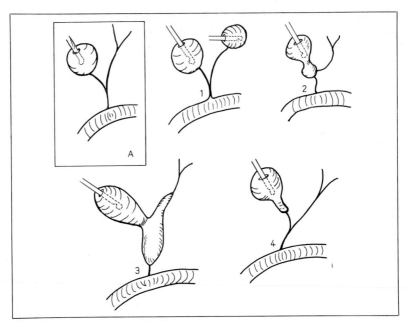

Fig. 2

patic region with no connection with the mentioned structures, which may permit an anastomosis with the intestine. In all the cases belonging to this type A, there is no passage of the contrast material into the intrahepatic branches or into the duodenum.

Type B includes cholangiograms where the contrast material passes through a rudimentary bladder into the cystic duct and to the common bile duct reaching the duodenum [fig. 3, copied from HAYS *et al.*, 1967, chap. 1].

In these types of cases, by clamping the common bile duct a certain repletion of the proximal hepatic system may be obtained with images that may correspond to the following types [fig. 4, copied from HAYS *et al.*, 1967, chap. 1].

Figures 2–4 are self-explanatory. Some pertinent details are stressed: In type E there is total repletion of only one of the hepatic branches. In type F, corresponding to the majority of cases, the branches may be identified only be enlarging the images. Type G corresponds to a 'normal' cholangiogram, with easy passage of the contrast material to the duodenum and with complete repletion of the extrahepatic and intrahepatic ducts.

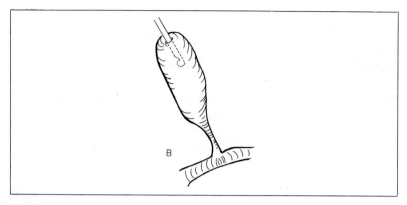

Fig. 3

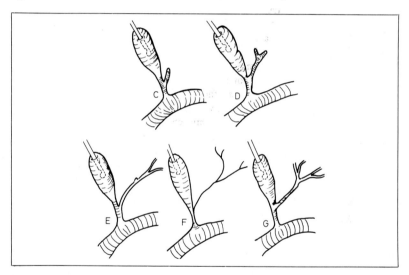

Fig. 4

Nevertheless, a careful observation in such cases may disclose the presence of irregularities with small regmentary dilations in the ducts; some of these cholangiograms reveal also a slight narrowing of the ducts and do not show the smooth edges of a totally normal image. Thus, this image is, at least in part, 'somewhat' pathological. These facts suggest that cases included in the triad, and considered as hepatitis, also show injuries of the external excretory ducts. No doubt this fact possesses a relevant significance in the concept of the 'inflammatory and atresia-inducing disease of the liver and bile ducts', the leitmotiv of this work.

From the study of the cases of the authors, the cholangiographic images are said to correspond to: (1) Type A: *almost always to atresia*, and in a few cases to hepatitis. Out of 17 cases with this type of image, the definitive diagnosis was of atresia in 16 and of hepatitis in one. (2) There are types that *always* indicate hepatitis, such as type G and perhaps also type F (although the number of observations is too small to give a definite classification). (3) There are some types, especially types B and C, that may correspond *either to atresia or hepatitis*. (4) The very few cases that give images of types D or E correspond to hepatitis.

Within the HAYS et al. [1967, chap. 1] classification there is not an explicit account of those cases with a nonpatent cystic duct, i.e. those in which the radiopaque contrast material does not go further than the gallbladder. This fact can be due to: (1) the existence of a true atresia of the cystic duct; (2) a lack of visualization of this duct, because it is occluded by exudates or excreted material[9]; (3) a technical defect. Obviously, there is not a mandatory correspondence between the cystic atresia and the patency of the main biliary channels (hepatic and/or common bile ducts). In fact, in the course of the surgical exploration, it is difficult to ascertain the patency of these structures, as it is not a sound practice to manipulate them, much less to puncture or to attempt to biopsy them. Nevertheless, with all likelihood, when the cystic duct is not patent and there is a small gallbladder containing no bile (cases 12 and 15, pp. 225 and 227), the main bile channels must be wholly or partly atresic. On the contrary, when the gallbladder appears fairly normal, or somewhat diminished in size, and it contains green bile, the patency of the main biliary ducts is most likely; failure of filling the ducts with the radiopaque substance must be explained by the above-mentioned causes (2 and 3) (case 11, p. 223).

In summary, the cholangiogram is not infallible to establish a distinction between hepatitis and atresia. The degree of diagnostic precision provided by this exploration reaches 79% of cases; in the other 21% the diagnosis is equivocal (8%) or erroneous (13%), according to the same authors.

C. Surgical Biopsy of the Liver

The large size of the sample obtained makes it more valuable than that obtained by needle biopsy.

Basing our experience mostly on surgical hepatic biopsies, we have gathered in table III, as a differential diagnosis, the histopathological characteristics of each one of the entities of the triad having reached a period of state; the elements that are classically considered as most out-

9   Favored by the tortuous course of this structure.

Table III. Microscopic pathology of the liver of each entity of the triad

Structural element	Extrahepatic atresia	Neonatal hepatitis	Intrahepatic atresia
Alteration of trabecular configuration:	little or none	■ severe	little or none
Cholestasis	■ *not limited to the lobule*	*limited to the lobule*	limited to the lobule with center lobular preference
Ducts = cholangioles	sometimes increased	normal or decreased in number	■ *decreased* or absent
Ductules = canals of Hering	■ usually clearly increased	may be increased	sometimes, clearly increased
Bile pigment content in:			
Ducts	■ often present and of great diagnostic value	–	–
Ductules	very often	sometimes	sometimes
Canaliculi (bile capillaries)	often	often	with great frequency
Hepatocytes	no distinctive features		
Presence of giant cells	quite often	■ very often	sometimes
Inflammatory cellular infiltration	without distinctive characteristics		in this entity, with periductal preference
Grouping in tubes or acini	+	+ +	■ + + +
Fibrosis	begins in the portal spaces; clear limitation of portal parenchymal space for a long time	from the beginning perilobular and lobular	perilobular and lobular; sometimes primary biliary cirrhosis
Hemopoetic foci	without distinctive characteristics		
Other altered elements	■ portal arteries increased in number and thickness	–	–

standing in each entity are indicated by a black square. For the sake of precision, the current terminology of the hepatic structures must be reviewed.

D. Terminology of Hepatic Structures

The nomenclature of the hepatic structures has been considered in a very specific manner in the 1962 Meeting of the New York Academy of Sciences on 'Fetal and Infant Liver Function and Structure'. In this conference, an agreement was reached in the definition of the following terms: *Tubule,* according to HORTSMANN [1969], signifies an embryonic element of the excretory system. *Ducts* are the already developed excretory structures. Some are extrahepatic (hepatic, cystic, common bile duct that together with the bladder constitute the principal bile duct); others are intrahepatic, whose terminal part, the smallest, is the portal duct, the interlobular duct, one of the three constituent elements of the small portal spaces of Kiernan. *Canaliculus* is the bile capillary, i.e. the excretory structure situated within the lobule and formed by the liver cells themselves.

No nomenclature agreement was reached on the following points: The *part of the excretory structure* located between the portal duct and the canaliculus. To WILSON [1963], following BLOOM and FAWCET [1964], it should be termed *cholangiole,* whereas POPPER and SHAFFNER [1957, chap. 1] and HOLLANDER and SHAFFNER [1968, chap. 1] prefer calling it *ductule.* This cholangiole or ductule corresponds to the portion also known as perilobular duct, intercalate channel or segment, or Hering's canal, according to the general consensus, but the canal of Hering, according to the image given of it by its author, really corresponds to the preductule, as on one end it continues with the hepatic cells and on the other with the ductule [WILSON, 1963]. In their work, STEINER and CARRUTHERS [1961] have already considered the canal of Hering as equivalent to the preductule.

Nevertheless, to call Hering's canal to the perilobular duct or ductule is such a widespread practice that, for the sake of general understanding, we are necessarily compelled at present to accept it. And if we define the ductule as the duct segment between the canaliculus and the portal duct, we will logically have to classify as preductule the most initial part, which joins the canaliculus.

Terminology that has become doubtful or equivocal: For a long time, authors have assigned *canaliculus* to the intralobular excretory structures, the bile capillary, located within the liver and formed by the hepatic cells themselves. But with increasing frequency this term has come to be understood as meaning the perilobular duct. From this originates, for example, the term used by several French authors, of 'neo-canalicule', applied to the proliferation of ducts that occurs in the portal spaces in secondary biliary cirrhosis. Yet these structures do not stem out from the real canaliculi but, at least for their greater part, from the ductules.

From what has been said, we infer that either the term canaliculus is ratified, reserving it only to designate the intralobular excretory structure, or we apply to this structure the new coined term 'capillicule' (currently used in recent French medical literature). This means 'small capillary'; the perilobular and interlobular ducts are really bile capillaries too, like the blood and lymphatic capillaries, their wall consists of a single layer of cells.

For a long time, *cholangiole* has been applied to the duct portion situated between the canaliculus and the chief septal ducts, and even now SHERLOCK [1971] uses it with this meaning.

From this follows that the term 'cholangiolitis' corresponds to an inflammation of these small ducts as opposed to that of cholangitis which designates an inflammation of the large extrahepatic and intrahepatic ducts. It can be seen then, that following WILSON [1963] and BLOOM and FAWCET [1964], by cholangiole we mean the intercalar portion between duct and canaliculus (or capilliculus). This can give rise to confusions with other terms which are already solidly rooted in the terminology of the hepatic structures.

Necessary ratifications of some terminological expressions: For the sake of precision it must be understood that: (1) The term *duct* is a generic expression that in a wider sense means an excretory structure, i.e. a channel through which the bile circulates from the origin of the canaliculus to the end of the common bile duct in the duodenum. For this reason, in connection with ducts, we must consider as 'perilobular' the ductule and reserve the term intralobular to designate both the preductule and the canaliculus. Nevertheless, in a strict sense, 'duct' has a more precise meaning, as previously defined above. (2) The term *canal* signifies any excretory structure of greater size located beyond the canaliculus; the definition of perilobular canal should be accepted, then, as very suitable for the designation of the ductule. (3) It would seem very logical to call *preductule,* as many authors do, the small initial portion of the ductule that merges into the canaliculus. (4) *Limiting plates* are the hepatic cells at the periphery of the lobule, bordering with the connective tissue, and are related at the extremes with the preductules.

From what we have said, it is apparent that there is a lack of uniformity regarding the concepts and terminology of the liver structures; the widely known and often quoted book by HAM [1969] has added much to this confusion. Actually, on p. 730, when dealing with certain structures, and according to electron microscopic studies by STEINER and CARRUTHERS it says:

'The canals of Hering along their short courses are borded in part by hepatocytes and in part by a different kind of cell which is not a secretory hepatocyte but a duct type of cell . . . The canals of Hering are very short and connect with the bile ductules (the finest branches of the bile duct system); these are present in the connective tissue of the portal radicles. However, the canals of Hering are not the only channels by which bile from canaliculi reaches the bile ductules in the portal radicles, because leading off at angles from the canals of Hering there are little bypasses which are termed preductules, and these too drain into the bile ductules that are in the portal tracts. Preductules differ from canals of Hering because they have no hepatocytes along their courses; their walls are made entirely of cells of the duct type. The walls of the preductules are seen to consist of no more than two or three cells of the duct type. The bile ductules (small bile ducts) in the portal tracts into which both the canals of Hering and the preductules drain, seen in cross section, have more than 3 cells around their walls. The bile ductules are merely the smallest branches of the branching tree of the bile ducts that is contained in the connective tissue tree, which sends tis branches to the periphery of all liver lobules.'

Therefore, according to HAM [1969]: (1) the terms canals of Hering and ductule are not equivalent; (2) canals of Hering and preductule are not equivalent terms either, and (3) the small ducts of the portal spaces, associated to relatively small arteries and veins, are called 'ductules' by HAM [1969].

From this discussion, it is evident that a strict definition of concepts and a unified terminology of the liver structures are desperately needed. Failure in achieving this uniformity has undoubtedly contributed to a certain confusion in the understanding of the pathology of the liver and bile ducts, especially in the sphere we are considering, i.e. the triad.

1. Neonatal Hepatitis

The most outstanding characteristics are:

The presence of giant parenchymal syncytial or plasmodial cells, with multiple nuclei. Usually, they are irregularly distributed; more frequent in some areas, less in others, they show a slight tendency to prevail in the

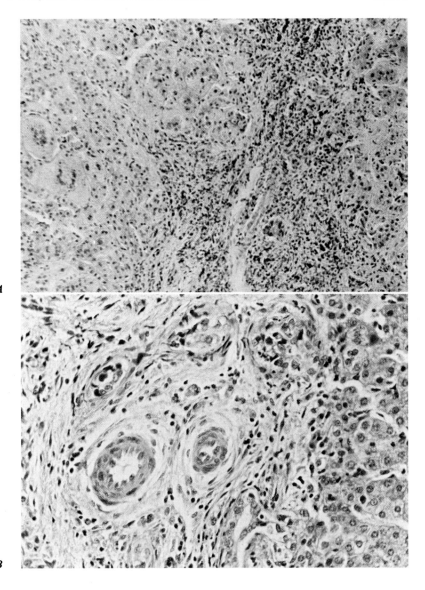

A

B

Cpl. I. Legend on reverse side of plate III.

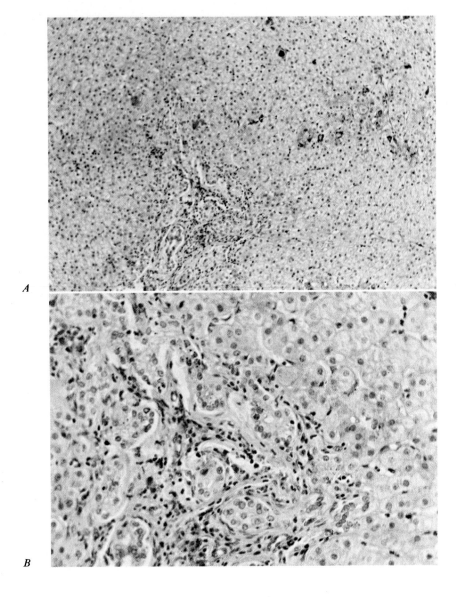

Cpl. II. Legend on reverse side of plate III.

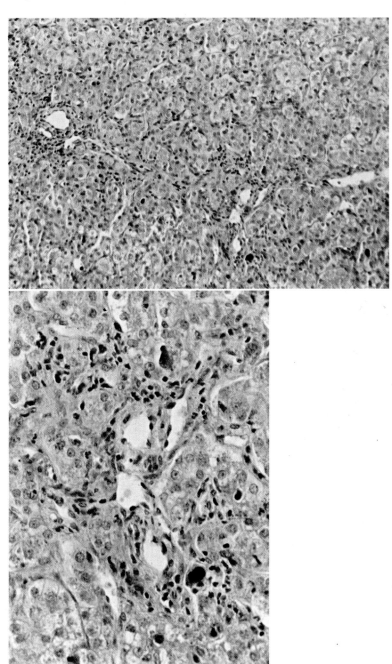

A

B

Cpl. III. Legend on reverse side.

The Inflammatory and Atresia-Inducing Disease

Legends for plate I–III

Cpl. I. A Neonatal hepatitis. Surgical biopsy specimen from a 3-month-old baby (case 1, p. 213). The case evolved to hepatic cirrhosis; the patient is now 12 years old and his condition is fair. Observation at low magnification. Zone with typical and extensive giant cell transformation of the hepatocytes; two adjacent ones show nuclei placed like a crown in one, clustered in its center in the other. Deep bile staining. Manifest trabecular disruption. Clear increase of the portal connective tissue and of the kupferian system and dense leukocytic infiltration in the connective spaces. *B* Extrahepatic atresia. Liver. Surgical biopsy obtained from an intervention carried out at the age of 55 days (case 4, p. 218). Marked fibrous portitis with moderate leukocytic infiltration. In the upper part, traces of three ducts with obvious signs of a degenerative process with decreased vitality; one of them contains a bile thrombus. In the central area of the picture, two arterioles with a wall thicker than usual; and, under them, next to the parenchyma, a better preserved bile duct.

Cpl. II. A Surgical liver biopsy in a case of extrahepatic atresia operated at the age of 3 months (case 3, p. 216). Towards the center of the lobule the pigmentation of the liver cells is quite obvious; pigment in some places forms small pool of bile. *B* Closer detail of *A*. Bile pigmentation can be demonstrated in the hepatocytes and cells of the ductules and ducts. In the remarkably fibrous connective tissue, macrophagic cells with phagocyted pigment are seen.

Cpl. III. A Surgical liver biopsy in a case of intrahepatic biliary atresia, with normal external ducts, confirmed by cholangiography (case 5, p. 218). Two spaces of Kiernan, one of them with considerable leukocytic infiltration and with no duct. *B* Detail of one of the two spaces of Kiernan in *A*. Note the great tubular transformation of the parenchyma; with the presence of thick bile thrombi in some of the tubules.

center and periphery of the lobule. If a giant cell offers a symplasmic aspect, it is because the section passes through a zone deprived of nuclei.

Changes in trabecular configuration, due to the great variation in the size of the cells (cpl. I) [CRAIG and LANDING, 1952].

The presence of multinucleated hepatocytes with giant cell transformation constitutes the most obvious feature in neonatal hepatitis, as pointed out by CRAIG and LANDING [1952]. Some authors classify it as 'neonatal hepatitis', especially because they doubt its inflammatory character. Although we later examine this point closely (p. 73), let us say at this stage: (1) that such syncytial cells are not consubstantial with neonatal hepatitis, because in many cases they are not present, and (2) that they can also be observed in other processes that are not even infectious (p. 51).

Along with the trabecular disorganization, obvious changes occur in the reticulin network which is missing (collapse of the reticule) in areas with giant cells, and increased in other areas, mainly due to greater thickness of the fibers. The framework of reticulin fibers will form a partition around the multinucleated cells.

2. Extrahepatic Biliary Atresia

Here, the most important microscopic features are:

1. Fibrosis of diverse intensity limited to the portal spaces for some time; only in advanced cases, a clear intralobular fibrosis is present.

2. A variable degree of proliferation of the bile ducts, particularly when it is not accompanied by intrahepatic atresia (fig. 5). This proliferation affects especially the ductule and the duct, and also the preductule, but probably with less intensity.

3. Cholestasis not limited to the lobule: bile, usually in large amounts, can be demonstrated within the ductular and ductal cells (cpl. II).

A bile retention reaching the ducts amounts to an almost pathognomonic sign of extrahepatic biliary atresia (cpl. IB).

4. Finally, an outstanding microscopic feature in extrahepatic atresia is an increase in the number and thickness of the portal arteries (cpl. IB).

3. Intrahepatic Biliary Atresia

The microscopic pathology of this entity is characterized by:

1. A marked decrease or even the absence of ducts, mainly in the connective spaces of Kiernan. That is in sheer contrast with the re-

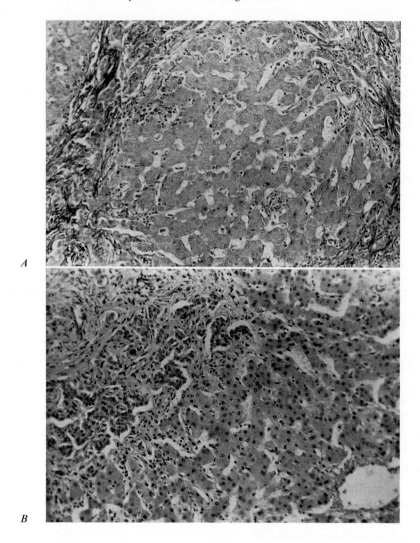

Fig. 5. A Microscopic view of the liver in extrahepatic atresia. Necropsy specimen of a patient who died in the 11th postoperative day, after 4 months of evolution of the disease (case 2, p. 215). Practically all the lobule is surrounded by fibrous tissue, with a very marked proliferation of biliary ductules and ducts. Only small bands of connective tissue penetrate into the lobule; the leukocytic infiltration is small. *B* Same patient as in *A*. Portal fibrosis and reduplication of biliary ductules and ducts. A bile thrombus can be seen within one of the ducts.

duplication, especially of the ductules, in certain places (cpl. XIB, XIIA). On occasion, the decrease in the number of ducts is not uniform but acquires a zonal character: regions with no ducts alternate with others where ducts are present in apparently normal numbers [BENAVIDES *et al.*, 1962, chap. 1].

2. According to our own observations, the disposition in acini or tubes of the hepatic trabecules which can also be observed in the other entities is much more patent in intrahepatic biliary atresia, occasionally lending the lobule a tubular structure (cpl. III).

III. Special Considerations on Certain Histopathological Features of Liver Biopsy Specimens

1. There is no constant or exclusive sign of an entity. The most valuable sign, which is considered by some authors as pathognomonic of extrahepatic atresia, is the presence of bile thrombi in the ducts. But the only pathognomonic fact in relation to the bile thrombi is that they evidence the presence of a downstream obstacle or blockade of the bile flow. We consider *almost* phathognomonic of extrahepatic atresia and of cases of intrahepatic atresia of the large ducts near the hilum, the presence of thrombi in the ducts of septa of a certain size, or its equivalent: a connective biliorrhagia due to fissure or destruction of the epithelium of these structures.

Almost pathognomonic, we insist, because they can also be due to other cholestatic processes which are certainly less frequent than atresia, and which block the responsible ducts, especially by external obstructive mechanisms.

We do not consider as valuable the presence of bile thrombi in the small ducts of the spaces of Kiernan or the little septa with two or three ducts. The bile thrombi so placed can correspond to intrahepatic atresia of the ducts of larger septa, which accompany the indicated atresia with more or less intensity, and that can also be seen in cases of hepatitis [CRAIG and LANDING, 1952; HANAI *et al.*, 1967; BROUGH and BERNSTEIN, 1969, chap. 1, and our own observations, cpl. VIA]. However, we also consider almost pathognomonic of extrahepatic and intrahepatic atresia of the large ducts near the hilum the bile thrombi found in small ducts or ductules of the periphery of a band of ductal-ductular and perilobular fibrous proliferation (cpl. IVA, VA) which are very characteristic in such cases of atresia or in cases of cholestasis of obstructive nature.

In consequence, there are certain limitations to the diagnostic value of the liver biopsy. A recent paper by HAYS *et al.* [1967, chap. 1] confirms this assertion; these authors consider the biopsy of a diagnostic value only in two thirds of the cases.

Furthermore, they state that the microscopic features of liver specimens in both diseases may offer a series of intermingled findings: (1) some cases of atresia present a greater quantity of giant cells than other cases of hepatitis; (2) the proliferation of the ducts which is taken as a characteristic sign of atresia is sometimes found in cases diagnosed as hepatitis; (3) biliary stasis of varying degree is found in both diseases, and (4) varying degress of cirrhosis can be present in both entities.

PICKETT [1962] observed several years ago that no decisive difference exists between cases that show a giant cell reaction either in hepatitis of diverse etiology or in cases with anatomical obstruction due to atresia.

The following cases are examples of the difficulties encountered in distinguishing hepatitis from atresia.

The first one, reported by DANKS and CAMPBELL [1966], is a case of incomplete 'icteric syndrome' in which a needle biopsy obtained at 5 weeks of age was interpreted as compatible with 'neonatal hepatitis'. Once the icteric syndrome became complete, at the age of 4 months, a cholangiography and a surgical biopsy were carried out. The pathological report was 'neonatal hepatitis'. At $5^1/_2$ months, the autopsy revealed an atresia of the main hepatic duct, which had already been shown in the cholangiography. The two previous biopsies were then reexamined and this time, on handsight, signs of portal fibrosis and ductal proliferation which could have suggested an atresia were found. The authors concluded from this that too much value had been given to the giant cell transformation of the parenchyma and to the intralobular fibrosis.

A more recent case report by DANKS *et al.* [1968] is that of an infant jaundiced from birth, with nonacholic feces for 11 days; the needle biopsy was suggestive of neonatal hepatitis. At 4 weeks of age, the feces became completely acholic; at 9 weeks, a cholangiography was carried out showing a free passage of the contrast material to the duodenum, but without filling of the hepatic ducts.

A surgical biopsy continued to show signs more suggestive of 'neonatal hepatitis' than of a mechanic obstruction. Surgical exploration did not reveal any traces of the hepatic duct outside the liver or in the dissection of the vessels inside the gland. Therefore, once atresia has already been established, as confirmed beyond any doubt by the autopsy, the appearance of the liver is not *yet* clearly defined, as in the forementioned case, and does not allow more than an ambiguous diagnosis. We wish to stress the fact that the typical microscopic features of extrahepatic atresia take some time (several weeks or even months) to develop.

To DODERO *et al.* [1969], the biopsy reports have no other virtue than to cloud the issue. According to these authors, these reports are hardly ever in agreement with the cholangiographic data and the operative findings. Furthermore, the microscopic diagnosis of the same specimen studied by two pathologists has been on many occasions radically opposed.

From the preceding discussion, the limitations or difficulties of liver biopsy in the diagnosis of the three entities become evident. These problems will be reconsidered in this chapter (sect. VI).

2. A giant cell reaction leading to classify hepatitis as 'neonatal hepatitis' is of no diagnostic value. The mere presence of giant cells does not justify the definition of a separate entity, considering that the number of cases of neonatal hepatitis in which these cells are found is relatively small.

According to ALAGILLE [1965], they are only found in 20% of cases; STOWENS [1959, chap. 1] finds a giant cell transformation of the parenchyma only in 8% of the cases. Nor are there any differences in clinical or laboratory data in neonatal hepatitis with or without giant cells. CRAIG and LANDING [1952] already pointed out that perhaps the diagnostic significance attributed to the presence of multinucleated cells in their cases of neonatal hepatitis resembling atresia had been exagerated. Actually, in one third of the cases of atresia, giant cells are also found, although in less quantity; in some cases, these cells even constitute a predominant element. Other authors also confirmed this opinion: ALAGILLE [1965] found giant cells in 17% of atresic cases, and SILVERBERG et al. [1960, chap. 1] state that one third of their atresic cases show a giant cell transformation of variable intensity. KASSAI et al. [1962] note this feature in half of their cases. HAYS et al. [1967, chap. 1] hold a similar view, stating that in some cases of atresia, they find more giant cells than in some other cases of hepatitis. Our observations agree with these opinions.

Consequently, as a giant cell transformation occurs only in a limited proportion of cases of neonatal hepatitis, it follows that the presence of giant cells and the diagnosis of neonatal hepatitis should not be considered as equivalent. Moreover, entities of a well-defined etiology have been extracted from this neonatal hepatitis with or without giant cells, which is a sort of 'odds and ends box', and it has even been seen that non-infectious, dismetabolic processes could mimic it. It has been confirmed that this occurs in galactosemia [in a recent paper by ROSCHLAU et al., 1969] and ornithinemia [BICKEL et al., 1968].

3. Ductipenia. The absence of duct or ducts in the connective spaces, especially in the spaces of Kiernan, usually affecting several, or exceptionally all of them, constitutes a fundamental characteristic of intrahepatic atresia; but a certain ductipenia can also be present in the other entities. It must be pointed out that it is not always feasible to determine whether in a connective space the duct or ducts are missing or not. This leads us to consider two types of ductipenia: the real and the apparent (pseudoductipenia).

a. We talk about true ductipenia when the duct is missing or the number of ducts in the connective space is decreased. Such a ductipenia will offer no doubts in interpretation, and will be evident when it occurs in a connective space that permits a clear and unmistakable definition, i.e. with scarce or no signs of infiltration by edema or inflammatory cells.

b. When a connective space presents an edematous or cellular infiltration, *especially if it is very marked*, its structures and in particular the duct or ducts are on many occasions very difficult to define. The image can be misleading and the failure to identify such structures by histological staining methods may correspond to:

1. A pseudoductipenia, i.e. (a) with a duct still demonstrable by histochemical methods, that through a positive reaction with their substrate can evidence its enzymes (phosphatases, leucine aminopeptidase) or (b) with a duct *not* revealable by histochemistry due to a dystrophic functional defect of the structure.

That a dystrophy of the excretory epithelial component can provoke an evident dysfunction (partial or total loss of function) of this element, may be readily seen in a recent observation in our series (case 16, p. 229) where the biopsy revealed an extensive dysmorphy-dystrophy-necrobiosis of excretory channels (see p. 78), although many of them were still recognizable. In spite of the existence of a practically complete cholostasis (radioiodinated) rose bengal, 10.6% at 48 h, no alkaline phosphatase isoenzyme of the biliary ducts ('the alkaline phosphatase of cholostasis') could be demonstrated in blood.

2. A true ductipenia – although not visible, not evident, and which cannot be unquestionably demonstrated as the 'image' of this ductipenia, is identical to that of paragraph 1(b).

In summary, ductipenia can be unquestionably accepted only under the conditions described in paragraph a.

4. The ductules. In extrahepatic atresia, as indicated in the pathological differential-diagnostic list, the number of perilobular ducts or canals of Hering tends to be significantly increased. The number of ducts may also be increased; this ductular-ductal proliferation constitutes one of the most peculiar and most constant signs of such a type of atresia.

A marked ductular hyperplasia accompanied by a hypoplasia of the interlobular ducts seems to be a characteristic feature in children with congenital biliary atresia, according to KASSAI *et al.* [1962]. Such a hypoplasia is quite apparent when it affects the interlobular ducts in portal spaces somewhat larger than Kiernan's (which being the smallest portal space contains only one artery, one vein and one duct), as Kiernan's ducts are difficult to distinguish from the ductules.

The demonstration of such a hypoplasia or hypotrophy ($=$ dystrophy, as indicated in footnote 11) is a sign of damage to the excretory epithelial elements as we shall see in the chapter on histopathogenesis, and in our opinion constitutes an obvious indication of the existence of a destructive process due to an agent that directly causes the injuries that will lead to atresia (atrophy).

In a simple extrahepatic obstruction, as is the case in common bile duct cyst, this hypotrophy with degeneration of the intrahepatic excretory ducts can also be demonstrated; but only in a moderate degree and after a long evolution of the disease. KASSAI et al. [1962] point out that to pass a definite judgment on the state of these interlobular ducts, an extense biopsy is required; needle biopsies do not provide enough material. Even in intrahepatic atresia, in which the decreased number of ducts is a fundamental defining element the number of ductules may be increased. SCHMID [1965] indicates that both in atresia of the extrahepatic ducts and in atresia of the small interlobular ducts the proliferation of the intercalary segments of Hering, the ductuli, is *meist intensiv*.

Perhaps in all entities of the triad there are more canals of Hering than one could imagine. In fact, in every hepatic injury, as GILMAN et al. [1954] pointed out, FARBER [1956] and LÓPEZ [1956] confirmed, and POPPER et al. [1957] studied experimentally, the reactions which are produced exhibit some clusters of cells in the portal spaces which have to be interpreted as ductular cells. If initially they can be mistaken as inflammatory cells, later on they take the shape of lengthened cells, disposed in a row with a central lumen. These cells are phosphatase-positive, as are the cells of the ductules and ducts, differing from the hepatic cells in that the latter are not phosphatase-positive, and that they surround a space which can be injected with contrast material (e.g. indian ink).

All hepatic injuries show an interstitial infiltration by inflammatory cells and mainly organized or disorganized ductular cells, that may even form channels. This reaction takes place in all animal species, even in humans, proceeds from the plates of the liver cells (liver cells in the periphery of the lobule), and can contribute to the production of granulomata, e.g. those of tuberculosis.

The perilobular ducts will therefore be identified with difficulty if they are not well organized, as they can offer the appearance of a ductular reaction very easily mistaken for an inflammatory one, especially of the fibroblastic type. As a result, and with the exception of cases of unequivocal ductular hyperplasia, we should consider here the existence of a true, but not evident ductular hyperplasia overshadowed by the inflammatory reaction. Histochemistry can identify some of these cases (demonstrable, nonvisible ductular hyperplasia) but other cases are not identified *(non*demonstrable, nonvisible ductular hyperplasia). In ductular hyperplasia, we believe that only rarely will a reaction falsely appear to be of the ductular type; such cases would fall into the category of *pseudoductular hyperplasia.*

5. Surgical biopsy. Although valuable diagnostic information can be obtained from a needle biopsy specimen of the liver, it is unquestionable that surgical biopsy, especially if taken from more than one zone, has a greater diagnostic value.

HAYS *et al.* [1967, chap. 1] have praised the diagnostic possibilities of the needle biopsy; STOWENS [1966] is of the same opinion and, based on the fact that the excretory structures are not distinguishable in the acute phase, he performs two needle biopsies. The first biopsy is taken at three weeks of age. (Incidentally, this is not usually done, because these patients are admitted to the hospital with considerable delay; on a clinical basis and with a limited number of laboratory examinations, a diagnosis of viral hepatopathy is usually assumed and a symptomatic therapy instituted.) The second needle biopsy is taken some weeks later.

A number of authors, however, consider the needle biopsy to have limited possibilities. In a survey carried out by the Surgical Section of the American Academy of Pediatrics in 1964 [IZANT *et al.,* 1964], it was revealed that many pediatricians never use puncture biopsy to differentiate atresia from hepatitis.

However, some authors still assign a great value to this method, considering that its diagnostic precision is similar to that of the surgical biopsy; in both cases, according to HAYS *et al.* [1967, chap. 1], a correct diagnosis can be established in two thirds of the cases. GENTILE-RAMOS [1970] reports 65% of correct diagnosis by needle biopsy in 'pseudomalformative' jaundices. The proportion of errors, nevertheless, according to HAYS *et al.* [1967, chap. 1], is clearly greater for needle biopsy (24%), than for surgical biopsy (9%). Inversely, the figures for the possibility of an equivocal diagnosis are 16% for puncture biopsy and 29% for surgical biopsy.

SHARP *et al.* [1967b, chap. 1] conceed only limited value to the needle biopsy for the purpose of establishing a diagnosis of ductipenia, as in the cases observed by them the large and middle-sized ducts are missing; the interlobular and the perilobular ones are present, though in smaller numbers.

It is our opinion that the limitations inherent to the needle biopsy, apart from the diagnostic difficulties that the microscopic diagnosis of the entities of the triad offer, are mainly related to: (1) the small size of the fragment, and (2) the fact that there is a tendency to perform the biopsy in the ascending period of the illness, when it still has not reached the period of state.

6. The nonexclusivity and lack of constancy of the micropathological signs suggest that there can be cases in which characteristic features of two or even three of the entities are present. Furthermore, a similar microscopic appearance can actually correspond to a different entity. This possibility was already pointed out some years ago. SILVERBERG *et al.*

[1960, chap. 1] observed cases studied by surgical biopsy, where the microscopic appearance is so imprecise that it can sometimes lead to false diagnoses, quite different from the clinical disease: cases of extrahepatic atresia which show microscopic signs typical of the liver in neonatal hepatitis. This has led many authors to stress the need for the pediatrician and the surgeon to realize that both diseases can be present together (extrahepatic atresia and neonatal hepatitis with giant cell transformation) and that microscopical observation by itself cannot be used to rule out atresia. The case reported by DANKS et al. [1968], quoted on p. 55, confirms SILVERBERG et al.'s [1960, chap. 1] point of view.

The intercorrelation of microscopic signs among the entities, and especially the 'substitution' of a typical image by another, as we have just mentioned, constitute very relevant aspects of the hepatic microscopic pathology of the entities of the triad. Out of them important logical foundations for the interpretation of their pathogenical determinism may be inferred.

IV. Diagnostic Value of the Hepatic Biopsy and
its Microscopic Features, According to our Concept

Following the synoptic list and the considerations we just made, it is possible to conclude that:

1. The surgical liver biopsy, especially when obtaining more than one fragment from different areas is of important diagnostic value although it should not be forgotten that only a very small and peripheric portion of the gland will be examined.

2. In extrahepatic atresia or intrahepatic atresia of the large ducts next to the hilum: (a) The presence of bile thrombi in septal ducts (i.e. ducts clearly separated from the periphery of the lobule) is of great diagnostic value. (b) The presence of bile thrombi in ducts and ductules in the periphery of a marked ductal-ductular proliferation with portal fibrosis is also of great diagnostic value. (c) A marked ductal-ductular proliferation with fibrous hyperplasia without thrombi, is also of significant diagnostic value.

The 'diagnostic value' of a microscopic feature should not be taken as an indisputable or an absolute clue to the diagnosis. In fact, the images indicated can also be secondary to an extrahepatic blockage due to causes other than atresia, i.e. intrinsic or extrinsic obstruction.

For the sake of maximal objectivity, we should add that a ductal proliferation can even be seen, although exceptionally, in cases of dysmetabolic jaundice producing hepatopathy, as is the case with galactosemia, where 'fatal cases were badly diagnosed as atresia, due to the histological image of ductal proliferation' [HARRIS, 1965]. As the existence of an extrahepatic blockage due to a cause other than atresia may sometimes be demonstrated only by direct or complementary explorations (cholangiography) of the ducts, a needle biopsy without information about the external structures of the liver allow us to make only a diagnosis of external blockage. Such a diagnosis will call for an immediate surgical exploration to confirm the diagnosis and to solve the blockage if feasible. If the efficiency of the exploration by means of the ultrasonic echo is confirmed, we will have the opportunity of diagnosing the cause of the blockage without having to resort to the operation.

3. In intrahepatic atresia: (a) A marked true portal and septal ductipenia of the small septs (containing normally at the most up to three ducts), higher than 50% with very few or no inflammatory signs (evident true ductipenia) is of great diagnostic value for pure or isolated atresia. (b) A marked apparent true ductipenia which includes the larger septa is of great diagnostic value for the association of intrahepatic with extrahepatic atresia.

4. In neonatal hepatitis: There are no elements of value to establish a microscopic diagnosis. This diagnosis can be provisionally accepted when the circumstances 2a, b, c, and 3a, b are not present; *but only provisionally,* awaiting the course of the microscopical examination, if it is deemed necessary. Only the natural evolution will say how the case will have to be classified – as hepatitis or atresia.

V. Diagnostic Value of the Combination of Cholangiography and Hepatic Biopsy

It has been clearly demonstrated that none of these methods alone permits one to reach a conclusive diagnosis.

The demonstration that cholangiography is not infallible seems, according to HAYS et al. [1967, chap. 1] to make the biopsy more important than it was before. The extensive simultaneous biopsy of both lobes through a laparotomy to reduce the sampling error resulting from small samples obtained from only one lobe can help in the diagnosis. The practice of repeated biopsies, at different times, can still increase the diagnostical possibilities. The above-mentioned authors obtained an incorrect diagnosis by cholangiography in three of their cases, whereas the hepatic biopsy provided a correct diagnosis of the disease, confirmed later on by the definitive diagnosis ['ultimate diagnosis' of HAYS *et al.*, 1967, chap. 1].

The combination cholangiography and hepatic biopsy has greater a diagnostic accuracy permitting a very probable diagnosis of an entity. According to data from the same authors, in 98% of the cases, one or another of the diagnoses was correct; only in 2% were both diagnoses wrong. Nevertheless, we must face the unavoidable dilema: which of the two diagnoses is correct?

When both diagnoses coincide, the problem would appear to be solved, except for this small 2% in which both are wrong. But, when they do *not* coincide, which should be accepted? This problem is dealt with in chapter 4.

We believe that besides this *very probable diagnosis* of an entity reached by combining the information gathered by cholangiography and liver biopsy, it is worth considering a high probability, *almost a sure diagnosis* of atresia which may be established in the following cases:

---

1. Extrahepatic atresia inferred from:
   a) Cholangiographic study and/or clinical findings presence of atrophic gall-bladder and ducts without bile
   b) Biopsy showing marked fibro-ducto-ductular proliferation plus bile thrombi and/or bilirrhages (cases 3, 13 and 15; pp. 216, 226 and 227)
2. Total atresia (extrahepatic and intrahepatic) inferred from:
   a) Cholangiographic study and/or clinical findings as in 1.a)
   b) Very marked true ductipenia and/or severe dysmorphy-dystrophy-necrobiosis process (cases 10 and 12, pp. 223 and 225)

VI. Further Considerations on the Contingencies of the Pathological Diagnosis by Means of Hepatic Biopsy

Having pointed out the limitations of the microscopic diagnosis, let us consider in greater detail this important point.

The diagnostic limitations of the biopsy depend mainly on two circumstances: on the existence of *mixed cases* and on the presentation of *particular cases* of diverse kind.

A. Mixed Cases

Mixed cases with microscopic features corresponding to more than one entity can exist due to the simultaneity or coincidence of the elements of two or three entities at the same time.

Table IV

Authors	Number of cases studied	Total atresia	Extrahepatic operable	nonoperable
LADD and GROSS	45	31	5	9
PROCHIANTZ	13	12	1	0
PETIT *et al.*	32	23	1	8
HESS	12	6	5	1

1. With the Elements of Two Entities
a) Extrahepatic and Intrahepatic Biliary Atresia

The association of extrahepatic and intrahepatic atresia was already pointed out by HESCHL [1865]. Although MOORE [1953, chap. 1] reported a rare incidence of this association (one mixed case among 19 of extrahepatic atresia), other authors' studies have demonstrated that actually such an association is a rather frequent observation.

AHRENS *et al.* [1951, chap. 1] in their review of 13 cases of intrahepatic atresia, found in 9 of them lesions of total or partial extrahepatic atresia. STOWENS [1966] states that extrahepatic atresia is accompanied by intrahepatic atresia in 10–15% of cases. SULAMAA and VISAKORPI [1964, chap. 1], in 41 cases of extrahepatic atresia, found the presence of intrahepatic atresia in 29. PILLOUD [1966, chap. 1], in his review of 56 cases of intrahepatic atresia, found 14 presenting extrahepatic atresia at the same time. A summary of a series of cases of extrahepatic atresia, reported by different authors, is shown in table IV [HESS, 1961].

It is here demonstrated that the simultaneous presence of both entities is quite common. The intrahepatic component has even been found in cases of familial extrahepatic atresia; this occurred in two of the three cases reported by SWEET [1932], where coexisting partial intrahepatic atresia was demonstrated.

b) Extrahepatic Biliary Atresia and Neonatal Hepatitis

Some cases reported by SCOTT *et al.* [1954], SILVERBERG *et al.* [1960, chap. 1], and DANKS and CAMPBELL [1966] were interpreted by these latter authors as possible instances of patients with two simultaneous illnesses. Nevertheless, if CRAIG and LANDING [1952] are right when pointing out that the presence of giant cells and the corresponding trabecular derangement are the most characteristic feature in hepatitis, the cases of extrahepatic atresia with giant cell infiltration mentioned by the authors should be considered in our opinion as a concomitance of atresia and hepatitis.

SMETANA et al. [1965] indicate that 21% of their cases of atresia exhibit a total or partial transformation of the hepatocytes into giant cells; SILVERBERG et al. [1960, chap. 1] raise this figure to one third; ALAGILLE [1965] points out its presence in 17% and STOWENS [1959, chap. 1] mentions an extensive transformation in 8% of his cases. In the new edition of his book, STOWENS [1966] classifies the giant cell transformation of the hepatocytes as an illness, stating that 20% of the cases of biliary atresia show it. These data prove the coexistence of both entities in the same patient to be very common.

c) Intrahepatic Biliary Atresia and Neonatal Hepatitis

The possibility of such association, indicated by SMETANA et al. [1965] can be readily accepted (p. 51). We have conclusively confirmed it in one of our cases of intrahepatic atresia showing a prominent giant cell transformation and trabecular distortion.

Similarly, one of our observations of neonatal hepatitis with a great quantity of syncythies showed bizarre images of dystrophy-dysmorphy-necrobiosis of the intrahepatic bile ducts, suggesting an evolution towards intrahepatic atresia that did not happen; the case healed, although with vestiges of a fibrosis and a moderate ductipenia. The child, who is at present 12 years old, has a normal biliary function, although a splenoportography has revealed a splenomegaly with decreased intrahepatic vascularization (case 1, p. 213).

2. Mixed Cases Presenting Microscopic Features of the Three Entities

Knowing there is a great number of cases of extrahepatic and intrahepatic atresia and a great proportion of cases of extrahepatic atresia with giant cell transformation, the possibility of observing microscopic features diagnostic of all three entities in a single case is readily acceptable.

In the literature, this possibility has not been considered. On logical grounds, it should not be a very exceptional contingency although it certainly could not be frequent either. One of our cases can be unquestionably considered, in our opinion, as an example of such an association, as the following microphotographs show (fig. 6).

B. Particular Cases

1. *Particular cases in relation with the evolutive moments.* For example, scarce fibrosis and ductal-ductular proliferation may be formed in cases of extrahepatic atresia of short evolution. THALLER and GELLIS [1968a–d, chap. 1] have pointed out recently that the process of fibrosis secondary to atresia of the external ducts does not undergo a notable development until the fourth month of postnatal life.

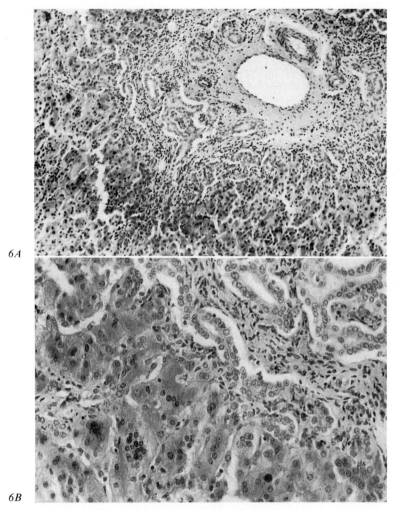

6A

6B

Fig. 6. A Surgical hepatic biopsy. Atresia of the external ducts in an infant operated at the age of 3 ½ months (case 6, p. 219). Large septum with ductular and ductal proliferation. No ducts offer a normal aspect according to the size of the septum. Note that in all of them the epithelium is low. *B* Greater detail of *A*. Note the abundant giant cell transformation. *C* Same case as *A*. Area with a large portal space where an arteriole and two other vessels can be clearly identified. The duct (or ducts) is missing. In the upper part of the portal space a zone of denser connective tissue with leukocytic elements is patent, suggesting that the interlobular excretory duct might have been located there. In this field, no giant cells or traces of ductal proliferation are seen. *D* Same case as *A*. A space of Kiernan with a clearly altered ductule is visible in the upper part; below is a remarkably dysmorphic duct. A very active giant cell transformation may also be noted.

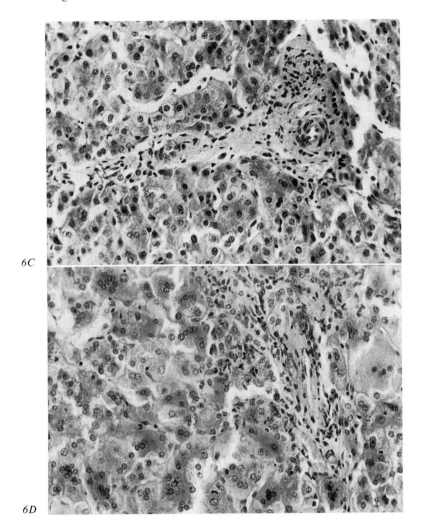

6C

6D

2. *Particular cases due to the extension or localization of the injuries.*
(a) Lack of fibrosis and ductal-ductular proliferation when there is a very
marked intrahepatic atresia concomitant with the extrahepatic form. (b)
Particular cases of patent external ducts with microscopic features of extrahepatic atresia (cpl. IV, VA), because atresia is localized in the great
intrahepatic ducts: in third degree [WILBRANDT, 1965, chap. 1] or second
degree [SMETANA *et al.*, 1965].

VII. Microscopic Pathology of the Triad: Conclusions

The existence of mixed cases and special ones leads us to these two important conclusions:

1. Hepatic biopsy has a recognized but restricted value in the diagnosis of each one of the entities. Necessarily, it will have to be correlated with the clinical and laboratory data and the liver function tests, especially the ^{131}I-rose bengal test, and occasionally with the surgical exploration with direct inspection of the biliary tree and operative cholangiogram. Only by using all this information can a practically certain diagnosis of each one of the entities of the triad be reached.

2. The mixed cases, which very often could be called transitory cases, and the special ones lead us to the logical inference, probably with a very small margin of error, that these three icteric processes of the newborn prolonged into infancy (extrahepatic biliary atresia, neonatal hepatitis, and intrahepatic biliary atresia) constitute diseases which are not independent from each other but narrowly interrelated. The following facts favor also this intercorrelation:

a) The pathologist may offer at times an unquestionable diagnosis, stating, for example, that extrahepatic atresia is accompanied in a great number of cases by intrahepatic atresia, or that in extrahepatic atresia, very often a component of neonatal hepatitis is found, which is expressed by the presence of multinucleated cells with the consequent trabecular disruption, etc.

b) In a number of cases the pathologist's diagnosis is wrong. As BAGGENSTOSS [1966] points out, it is easy and without risk for the pathologist to establish a symptomatic-morphological diagnosis, as for example, cholestasis, pericholangitis, fibrosis, etc., diagnoses that are of little help to the clinician. But when the pathologist ventures an etiological or pathogenical diagnosis based only on the microscopic study, a significant margin of error exists.

Thus, quoting BAGGENSTOSS [1966] in relation with extrahepatic obstruction (in adults), in 65 cases where such a pathogenic diagnosis was advanced by the pathologist, it was finally confirmed in only 54, or 83% of the cases. The causes of the error corresponded to intrahepatic diseases: cholangitis, hepatitis, etc.

But in other cases, the cause of error in the diagnosis lays in the fact that the clinical entity which is suspected and finally proved presents an abnormal and different microscopic appearance which entirely corresponds to another entity 'erroneously' diagnosed, as in the cases of SILVER-

BERG *et al.* [1960, chap. 1] and the case of DANKS *et al.* [1968]. What is *mistaken or erroneous in these cases is, one might say, the microscopic appearance.* These cases are, of course, much better understood if they are considered as mixed cases and belonging to the inflammatory and atresia-inducing disease, as we shall see later (chap. 3).

c) The most obvious proof of the close interdependence between the entities of the triad arises when considering the histopathogenesis of each one of them.

References

ALAGILLE, D.: Les ictères du nouveau-né. Pädiat. FortbildK. Praxis, vol. 15, p. 43 (Karger, Basel 1965).

BAGGENSTOSS, A. H.: Morphological and etiological diagnosis from hepatic biopsies without clinical data. Medicine, Baltimore *45:* 435 (1966).

BICKEL, H.; FEIST, D.; MÜLLER, A. und QUADRECK, G.: Die Ornithinemie, eine neue Aminosäure-Stoffwechselstörung mit Hirnschädigungen. Dt. med. Wschr. *93:* 2247 (1968).

BLOOM, G. and FAWCET, O. W.: Hystogenesis of the liver and its ducts. Textbook of histology, p. 487 (Saunders, Philadelphia, 1964).

CRAIG, J. M. and LANDING, B. H.: Form of hepatitis in neonatal period simulating biliary atresia. Archs Path. *54:* 321 (1952).

DANKS, D. M. and CAMPBELL, P. E.: Extrahepatic biliary atresia. Comments on the frequency of operable cases. J. Pediat. *69:* 21 (1966).

DANKS, D. M.; CLARKE, A. M.; JONES, P. G., and CAMPBELL, P. E.: Further comments on potentially operable cases. J. pediat. Surg. *3:* 584 (1968).

DODERO, P.; POSSENTI, B.; RIZZO, V.; GILLI, G.; GUSMANO, R. e MEZZANO, A.: Contributo statistico allo studio dell'atresia congenita delle vie biliari. Riv, Chir. Pediat. *21:* 313 (1969).

FARBER, E.: Similarity in the sequence of early histological changes induced in the liver of the rat by ethionine 2-acetylaminofluorane and 3′-methyl-4-dimethyl aminoazobenzene. Cancer Res. *16:* 142 (1956); cit. POPPER, KENT and STEIN.

GENTILE-RAMOS, I.: La punción biopsia del hígado en pediatría. Indicaciones y utilidad. Orbe Pediatrico No. 14, XI, p. 55 (1970).

GILMAN, J.; GILBERT, C., and SPENCE, I.: Some factors regulating the structural integrity of the intrahepatic bile ducts with special reference to primary carcinoma of the liver and vitamin A. Cancer *7:* 1109 (1954); cit. ELIAS.

GRAY, O. P. and SAUNDERS, R. A.: Familial intrahepatic cholestatic jaundice in infancy. Archs Dis. Childh. *41:* 320 (1966).

GUBERN-SALISACHS, L.: Personal Commun. (1970).

HAM, A. W.: Histology; 6th ed., p. 730 (J.B. Lippincott,, Philadelphia 1969).

HANAI, H.; IDRIS, F., and SWENSON, D.: Bile duct proliferation in atresia and related hepatic diseases. A morphological study. Archs Surg., *94:* 14 (1967).

HARRIS, J. H., jr.; O'HARA, A. E., and KOOP, C. E.: Operative cholangiography in the diagnosis of prolonged jaundice in infancy. Radiology 71: 806 (1958).

HARRIS, R. C.: Metabolic problems related to prolonged obstructive jaundice. 11th Int. Congr. Pediat., Tokyo 1965, p. 418.

HESCHL: Vollständiger Defekt der Gallenwege beobachtet bei einem 7 Monate alt gestorbenen weiblichen Kinde. Wien. med. Wschr. 15: 493 (1865); cit. MOY-SON, F.; GILLET, P. et RICHARD, J.: Agénésie des canaux biliaires intrahépatiques. Helv. paediat. Acta 8: 281 (1953).

HESS, W.: Die Erkrankungen der Gallenwege und des Pankreas; Spanish ed., p. 127 (Thieme, Leipzig 1961).

HORTSMAN, E.: Entwicklung und Entwicklungsbedingungen des intrahepatischen Gallengangssystems. Arch. Entwick. Mech. Org. 139: 364 (1969); cit. POPPER. KENT and STEIN.

IZANT, P. J., jr.; AKERS, D. R.; HAYS, D. M.; MACFARLAND, F. A., and WREN, E. L., jr.: Biliary atresia survey presented before section on surgery, Am. Acad. Pediatrics (1964); not published, cit. HAYS et al.

KASSAI, M.; YACOVAC, W. C., and KOOP, C. E.: Liver in congenital biliary atresia and neonatal hepatitis. Archs Path. 74: 152 (1962).

LLANIO, R. and JORDAN, J.: Laparoscopy and laparoscopic cholangiography in the diagnosis of prolonged obstructive jaundice in infants. 11th Int. Congr. Pediat., Tokyo 1965, p. 323.

LOPEZ, M.: Proliferazione iperplastiche e neoplastiche delle vie bilifere intrahepatiche da tiocetamide. Experientia 12: 143 (1956).

PICKETT, L. K.: in BENSON, MUSTARD, RAVITCH, SNYDER and WELCH Pediatric Surgery, p. 620 (Year Book Med. Publishers, Chicago 1962).

POPPER, H.; KENT, G., and STEIN, R.: Ductular cell reaction in the liver in hepatic injury. J. Mt Sinai Hosp. 24: 551 (1957).

ROSCHLAU, G.; AMKEL, G. K. and GOTSCHALK, B.: Klinische und morphologische Befunde zum Verlauf der Galaktosemie. Mschr. Kinderheilk. 117: 7 (1969).

SCHMID, M.: Zur diagnostischen Bedeutung der Leberpunktion in der Pädiatrie, Pädiat. FortbildK.Praxis, vol. 15, p. 31 (Karger, Basel 1965).

SCOTT, R. B.; WALKINS, W., and KESLER, A.: Viral hepatitis in early infancy. Report of 3 fatal cases simulating biliary atresia. Pediatrics, Springfield 13: 447 (1954).

SHERLOCK. S.: Diseases of the liver and biliary system, 4th ed., p. 703 (Blackwell, Oxford 1971).

SMETANA, H. F.; EDLOW, L. B., and GLUNZ, P. R.: Neonatal jaundice. Archs Path. 80: 553 (1965).

STEINER, J. W. and CARRUTHERS, J. S.: Studies of the fine structure of terminal branches of the biliary tree. I. The morphology of normal bile canaliculi, bile-preductules (ducts of Hering) and bile ductules. Am. J. Path. 38: 639 (1961).

STOWENS, D.: Diseases of the liver. Pediatric pathology, 2nd ed., p. 504 (Williams & Wilkins, Baltimore 1966).

SURUGA, K.; HIRAI, Y.; NAGASHIMA, K.; WAGAI, T., and INUI, M.: Ultrasonic echo examination as an aid in diagnosis of congenital bile duct lessons. J. pediat. Surg. 4: 452 (1969).

SUMMERSKILL, W. H. J.: The syndrome of benign recurrent cholestasis. Am. J. Med. *38:* 298 (1965).

SUMMERSKILL, W. H. J. and WALSHE, J. M.: Benign recurrent intrahepatic 'obstructive' jaundice. Lancet *i:* 686 (1959).

SWEET, L. K.: Atresia of the bile ducts. A report of three cases in one family. J. Pediat. *1:* 496 (1932).

SWENSON, O.: Personal Commun. to Silverberg *et al.* (1960) (see chap. 1).

SWENSON, O. and FISHER, J. H.: Surgical aspects of liver disease. Pediatrics, Springfield *16:* 135 (1955).

WILSON, J. W.: Discussion workshop. Terminology. Ann. N.Y. Acad. Sci. *111:* 513 (1963).

Chapter 3

Histopathogenesis of the Entities of the Triad

Taking as starting point the microscopic pathological injuries in their dynamic evolutive aspect, without taking into account their causative agent, the histopathogenesis of the triad is interpreted as follows:

I. Extrahepatic Atresia

This is an inflammatory process with notable parenchymal alteration affecting with preference the excretory epithelial system of the great external ducts, but usually without sparing the internal ones. It has the following distinct features:

1. Degenerative-Necrobiotic Process. This epithelial injury is accompanied constantly by a more or less intense infiltration, by cells and edema and by a connective tissue reaction which may be of the acute, subacute or chronic type, depending on whether the case is recent or of short or long evolution (fig. 7 and 8).

The total or partial destruction of the epithelium allows the production of a connective scar, initially with a variable infiltration by leukocytic elements, which later on will become fibrotic and eventually sclerotic if the evolution persists long enough; this scar tissue will replace the deteriorated structure. True atresia with total obliteration of the structure will result if the destruction reaches all the circumference of the lumen and there is no sign of epithelial regeneration.

If the 'atresying' process affects all the extrahepatic excretory structures, from the main branches of the hepatic duct to the duodenum, the result will be its conversion into mere cords, which are fibrous and hard. It seems that this pattern of evolution is quite rare. What usually happens is that the gallbladder or part of it is spared, resulting in a cavity of variable size. Sometimes, cavities or cystic areas may develop on the remnants of the ducts. When this occurs in the common hepatic duct or its main branches, and the cavity communicates with the intrahepatic ducts, the possibility for a successful bilio-intestinal anastomosis exists.

On other occasions, the destructive process does not affect all the circumference of the ducts or, perhaps, a partial regeneration takes place; in these cases a true atresia, in the etimological sense of the word, does not occur[10]. Part of the lumen has narrowed in an extension that varies with the length of the affected ducts. If the lesion is extensive and the ducts show very little or no function at all, due to the decrease or absence of choleresis caused by the associated hepatopathy, it can be understood that these ducts will appear scarcely developed or hypoplastic[11] as many authors describe them.

It seems that observations of this false atresia are not rare, although their actual incidence is not easy to establish, as those cases can only be adequately studied at the autopsy, since the external bile ducts should not be biopsied. However, the cholangiographic studies by HAYS et al. [1967, chap. 1] demonstrating on accasions rudimentary structures in the main bile duct, certify the existence of such cases. These authors agreee with RICKHAM's point of view that practically in all cases of atresia a rudimentary tract of the external ducts is found. The epithelial degenerative-necrobiotizing lesions reveal the existence of a destructive process affecting these structures and the observation in some places of well-developed traces of them constitutes indisputable proof that a deleterious cause acted after they had developed. These facts and, especially these cases which are erroneously diagnosed as atresia, evidence the great histopathogenic similarity between hepatitis and atresia.

In all cases of extrahepatic atresia where a fairly good extension of the parenchyma can be studied, it is usually possible to demonstrate a variable process of intrahepatic atresia. This might sometimes go unnoticed, especially if the liver fragment examined is very small, and the feel-

10   These cases cannot be labeled as partial or segmentary atresia, because atresia specifically means lack of lumen or patency in a duct. Partial or segmentary atresia would mean absence of lumen in part of the duct.

11   Nevertheless, we do not consider adequate the term of hypoplasia. We believe that *hypotrophy* or, even better, *dystrophy* would be more suitable and more specific while *still taking into account that this term only partially states what really happens to the structures (p. 78).*

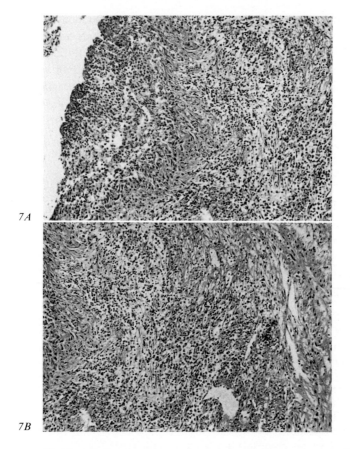

7A

7B

Fig. 7. A–D Extrahepatic atresia. Autopsy specimen corresponding to figures 5 A and B (case 2, p. 215). Section at the hepatic duct level, pairing off the slides: Subacute inflammatory process affecting nearly all the ductal wall, characterized mostly by connective proliferation and mononucleated leukocytic infiltration. The presence of remnants of

ing that the extrahepatic atresia is responsible for the clinical picture of the disease is already very strong. Furthermore, on many occasions the disease may offer 'contradictory' features, like signs of regeneration-*proliferation* of part of the excretory elements, mainly the ductules and in a smaller proportion the small ducts. The impulse responsible for such a regeneration-proliferation activity would appear to be the blockage of the bile. This problem will be discussed again later on.

It is very difficult to decide which of the two factors involved in the

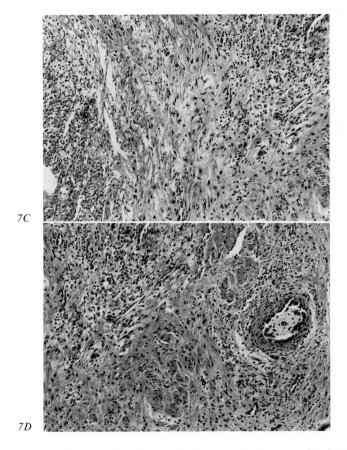

7C

7D

bundles of muscle fibers identify the fragment of tissue as belonging to a hollow organ although almost all its epithelial elements have disappeared. Only traces of the bottom of a crypt ballooned by blood and shedded cells from the superficial layer of devitalized epithelium.

histopathogenesis of atresia, i.e. obliteration and inflammation, is the leading one. As for the defective or absent structures, they could be explained by a developmental defect of the external excretory structures or by the action of a noxious agent after organogenesis is completed. The demonstration of well-developed structures (meta- or para-ontogenic, not orto-primo-ontogenic) with a normal or practically normal aspect (fig. 8B), may be offered as proof that an injuring agent, acting during the fetal period, is the principal if not the only cause.

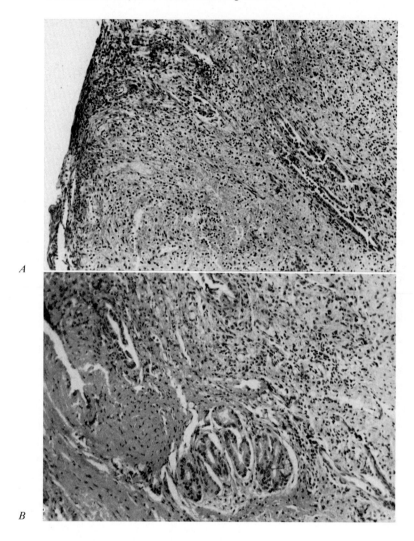

Fig. 8. A Case 2, as in figure 7 A–D. Atrophic-necrobiotic crypts and a surface deposit of fibrinous-leukocytic material may be seen. *B* A crypt of tubular glandular aspect surrounded by loose connective tissue, fairly well respected by the pathological process. Well-developed structures with no signs of hypogenesis.

Histopathogenetic Expression of the Obstacle to the Bile Flow

The impediment to the bile circulation produces three histological signs that deserve special consideration; the production of bile thrombi, the dilation of the ducts, and the ductule-ductal and connective proliferation. Let us now examine the first two of these signs in some detail.

a. Production of bile thrombi. The blockage of the bile flow is believed to be the main cause in the production of bile thrombi in the ducts, or of its equivalent, the connective biliorrhages due to the destruction of their epithelium; this is quite logical and already well known.

It is also common knowledge that this manifestation of extrahepatic atresia is not constantly observed. Nevertheless, it must be pointed out that an indicating element of the difficulty in the circulation of the bile in atresia is also represented by the presence of bile thrombi at the level of the ductules and small ducts near the parenchyma. It has been confirmed by electron microscopy studies [HOLLANDER and SCHAFFNER, 1968, chap. 1] that these structures show a capacity to absorb bile; the optical image itself allows us to demonstrate this fact (cpl. VA). But their absorptive capacity can be surpassed and bile may then be retained in their lumina. Nevertheless, bile is totally or almost totally reabsorbed into the ductules or ducts that are found further on, because neither the lumen nor the cells of these ductules or ducts show the presence of bile.

Interpretation and significance of the bile thrombi depending on their situation: (1) The bile thrombi situated in the ductules and small ducts near the trabecules, as all the evidence indicates, may be due to the bile elaborated by the lobule which is situated in their immediate proximity; as this bile may not flow on, it is absorbed by the ductule-ductal cells, from which it passes to the connective tissue and to the lymph or blood vessels. (2) It is more difficult to determine the origin of the bile thrombi situated in the ductule-ducts of the external zone of the ductule-ductal proliferation. The fact that such thrombi are situated in a band beyond a zone without thrombi seems to indicate that they are due to the reflux or back flow of bile from other zones, from ducts of larger caliber. Nevertheless, the fact that these ducts of larger caliber do not contain bile, especially if they are atresic, suggests that such thrombi can be due to the bile from immediate lobules that was not reabsorbed. Whatever the mechanism of its origin, it may be ascertained, given its greater or totally verdinic character, that its origin is older than that of bilirubin thrombi (cpl. IVA, VA).

b. Dilation of the supraatresic ducts. Cystic cavities of variable size, often deprived of epithelium and with signs of reabsorption of the pigment, can be observed in extrahepatic atresia.

It seems that the production of cystic cavities should be quite obvious and evident. It is surprising, however, that this does not commonly occur. On the contrary, as DANKS [1965, chap. 1] has repeatedly pointed out, the supraatretic dilation is always slight; it becomes more clear (but not very marked) in cases with a long course. On this delayed dilation of the ducts is based this author's idea that the longer the course of a case of atresia the greater its chances of operability, as the intrahepatic dilations of the biliary tree near the hilum will allow to perform an anastomosis. Note that an increase in the number of operable cases does not necessarily signify a parallel increase in the number of curable cases.

1. It is difficult to explain why the supraatresic ducts do not dilate more frequently and more markedly; we are not able to single out a cause as chiefly responsible. According to our point of view, contributing factors might be the limited bile secretion during the last part of the fetal period and the beginning of extrauterine life, the regurgitation of the bile which cannot travel easily through the canaliculus via the blood and lymph vessels, and the retention in the hepatocyte itself. Perhaps the reabsorption at ductule and small duct level plays a significant role.

2. The fact that cases which have become operable are not curable (i.e. by means of a bilio-intestinal anastomosis) could be explained, we believe, by the presence of devitalized and partially destroyed epithelium lining the dilated ducts. Actually, the epithelium is still submitted to the action of the morbid agents for a period of time after the operation. The healing of the process does not depend merely on providing a drainage to the bile flow, but especially on the immunobiological conditions of the macroorganism, when it overcomes or destroys the responsible agent. The possibility of achieving an efficient and lasting anastomosis depends intrinsically on a favorable outcome in the battle against the noxious agent and on the capacity for regeneration of the structures. It should be quite clear then that the dilation of the supraatresic bile tree does not correspond to a simple bile accumulation in ducts with a healthy and complete epithelial lining. It is the result of bile stasis in structures that are already diseased or will become altered (cpl. VB).

We do not share the opinion voiced by GREWE [1964] and SZENTPÉTERY [1964] and accepted by WELTE [1971] that failure of a bilio-enteric anastomosis should be explained on the basis of a quick growth of the connective tissue and the mucous membrane at the anastomotic opening. We believe that the patency of an anastomosis cannot be maintained if its epithelial lining fails to thrive or fails to adequately regenerate; this would show its involvement in a degenerative d-d-n process (p. 78).

c. Bile retention is mainly responsible at least for a ductular-ductal and connective proliferation process which we consider below.

2. Ductular-Ductal and Connective Proliferation

The inflammatory-destructive process is accompanied by regenerative phenomena, usually not very apparent on deteriorated structures. In a good number of cases of extrahepatic atresia, a clear ductal and specially ductular proliferation may be demonstrated at the intrahepatic level.

There is no doubt that the ducts participate to a certain extent in such a proliferation. The proliferated ducts situated deep inside the connective tissue (of the portal spaces and above all the septal ones) do not appear to correspond to anything else but ducts. But in such cases the cellular structure would appear to be also of 'ductular' type, as color plate XIVA seems to prove, and the existence of a process of dedifferentiation in such a ductal proliferation is either involved, or is simultaneous with it. An already mature, or relatively mature epithelium, with a definite shape and excretory duct function, has receded into a structure ontogenically younger, functionally more immature, and with greater capacity for proliferation.

It is not easy to decide the intrinsic cause of such a proliferation, although the retention of bile, as we already mentioned, and the greater cellular reproductive capacity that accompanies dedifferentiation, seem to constitute the most important elements of its determinism. Bile retention would act simply by irritating the epithelium or stimulating it to perform a greater resorptive action as an expression of a functional excitation. The fact that bile retention constitutes a very important element, probably the main one, of ductule-ductal proliferation, has been recently confirmed by BROUGH and BERNSTEIN [1969, chap. 1] who found a very marked proliferation in cholestasis due to obstruction of the external ducts, specifically in the case of a cyst in the common bile duct. Likewise, it is already known that the experimental ligation of the excretory ducts is accompanied by a prompt ductular proliferation. STEINER et al. [1962] find, in rats, that the first histological sign of interruption of the bile flow is ductular proliferation, soon accompanied by alteration of the vascular bed, with granulation tissue surrounding the ductules.

Whatever the intrinsic cause of such a regeneration-proliferation, it constitutes an element of great interest and importance in the histopathogenesis of extrahepatic atresia and also of the other entities; this is further discussed in section VI (this chapter).

Considering extrahepatic atresia in its dynamic evolutive aspect, its histopathogenesis shows the image of fibrosclerosis, giving the liver the characteristics of secondary biliary cirrhosis.

II. Neonatal Hepatitis

From the histopathogenetic point of view, most cases of neonatal hepatitis appear as an acute or subacute inflammatory process, while other cases have a chronic appearance with vascular-connective reaction and leukocytic infiltration. There is also a parenchymal alteration with a well-known feature consisting in the transformation of the hepatocytes into multinucleated elements (cpl. VI, fig. 9A and B).

A. Nature of the Giant Cells

The nature of these giant cells continues to be a matter of controversy. While many authors have considered them as cells that represent an attempt at regeneration, others interpret them as a degenerative manifestation. Some authors find a positive Fe reaction while others describe a negative reaction. Some mark its glycogen contents, others do not find it.

For some authors, they have been more or less specific indicators of the diagnosis. To many authors, the expression 'hepatitis with giant cells' means more than a pathological entity.

Very similar, if not identical cells, have been found in a good number of diseases: syphilis, hemolitic anemia [CRAIG and LANDING, 1952, chap. 2], etc. even in dysmetabolic illnesses; in many diseases in which there is a cellular degeneration and regeneration. This has led some authors to classify such cells as the nonspecific answer of the small infant to numerous stimuli of diverse nature.

Nevertheless, ATERMAN [1963] does not agree with this interpretation. To him it is difficult to understand why the liver of the infant only occasionally responds to nonspecific noxious agents; e.g. such cells are not observed in the toxoplasmosis of the newborn, in the diseases due to the Coxsakie virus, and they are not regularly seen in cytomegalic infection or in disseminated herpes simplex.

Observations carried out following ATERMAN's [1963] concept have allowed the demonstration of the fairly frequent presence of multinucleated elements in diseases in which they had only rarely been found before, e.g. in cytomegaly [WELLER and HANSHAW, 1962].

In summary, we can conclude that the presence of giant cells is so variable and they are present in processes of such different nature that their appearance will logically have to be considered as mainly dependant on a certain age, probably the first stages of extrauterine life (the opinion is unanimous in this respect), and on certain individual characteristics. Such a concept is sustained by the fetus-neonatal hepatopathy produced by a well-known virus that is held to be the causal agent of hepatitis and atresia: the rubella virus. Some authors [SINGER et al., 1967] have described cases of hepatitis without giant cells; others [ESTERLY et al. 1967], with them, and STRAUS and BERNSTEIN [1968] have found multinucleated cells in some cases of atresia and hepatitis but not in others.

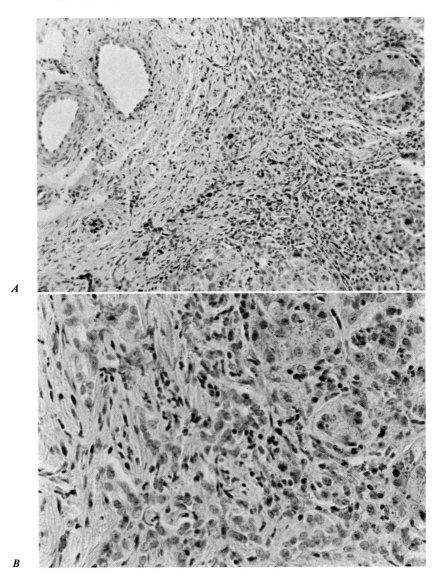

A

B

Cpl. IV. Legend on reverse side of plate VI.

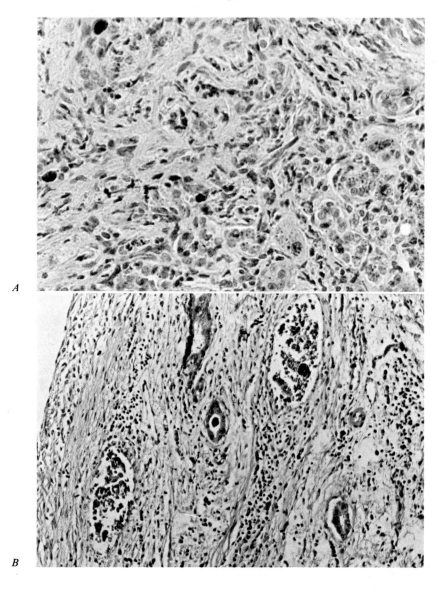

A

B

Cpl. V. Legend on reverse side of plate VI.

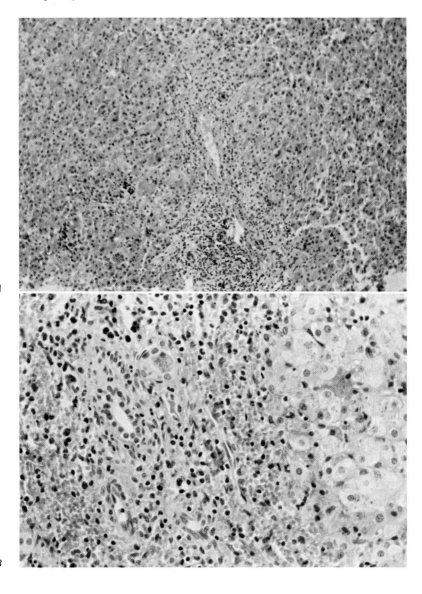

A

B

Cpl. VI. Legend on reverse side.

The Inflammatory and Atresia-Inducing Disease

Legends for plate IV–VI

Cpl. IV. A Atresia of the great ducts near the hilum. Surgical biopsy obtained at 4 ½ months of age (case 7, p. 220). Very marked ductule-ductal and fibrous proliferation. Abundant, newly formed ducts and ductules, with bile staining of those situated nearest to the hepatocytes. In the ducts situated in the periphery of this proliferation, two bile thrombi are clearly distinguishable. Beyond the proliferation zone, within a network of lax connective tissue, the outline of a degenerated devitalized septal duct with a lumen occupied by cell remnants may be identified in the lower left section of the picture. *B* Part of *A* at greater magnification. Marked proliferation of the channels apparently corresponding to ductules. Some elements with marked bile staining might be classified as preductules; the morphology is tubular, not trabecular, and the cells are not cubic but clearly prismatic, with a good number of elongated nuclei.

Cpl. V. A Detail of color plate IV A at greater magnification. (1) At the lower left, some hepatic cells and a good number of ductules with rubinic bile content in the form of intraluminal thrombi and granules phagocyted by the cells. In a duct further up, bile granules are found in the higher cells and near them there is a polynuclear leukocyte with a bile granule. (2) On the right of the image, two bile thrombi of verdinic appearance are seen within a ductal lumen. (3) Towards the center of the image and a little lower down, a fairly devitalized duct with three small thrombi: two smaller ones which are rubinic, and a larger one clearly verdinic, are noted. *B* Atresia of the external ducts at autopsy observed at the cystic-hepatic junction and in the common bile duct, in the extraintestinal portion; with a moderate cystic dilation of the hepatic duct near the hilum and with pronounced dilations in the large intrahepatic branches (case 15, p. 227). Section at the level of the large biliary intrahepatic ducts. Next to various ducts with epithelium affected by a process of degeneration and necrobiosis, three cystic cavities can be seen; one, to the left of the image not covered by epithelium or endothelium; another two in the middle of the retained biliary material (for further details, see case report).

Cpl. VI. A Neonatal hepatitis. Surgical biopsy at 4 days of age (case 8, p. 221). Extensive and intense inflammation with marked vascular reaction and pronounced cellular infiltration. Small septal space with two sections of a vein; the one on the upper part is clearly dilated; near it is a devitalized duct containing a bile thrombus. The duct is separated from the periphery of the lobule by two layers of fibroblasts; between one of them and the parenchyma is coagulated plasma or fibrine. In the lower septal portion, clear ductal proliferation among dense leukocytic infiltration (see detail in cpl. XI B). Evident bile staining of the hepatocytes, some of them are transformed into giant cells, as shown in colorplate VI B and figure 9A, B. *B* Septal space and perilobular zones. Good number of hepatocytes with eosinophilic protoplasm. Some show condensed or frankly pycnotic nuclei. On the right of the image, near the edge, a giant cell with two marginated pycnotic nuclei. Two ducts are clearly visible in a large portal space. One of them cut lengthways, with a vast lumen and low, cubic epithelium, with a certain irregularity in some of its nuclei, expression of an obvious although moderate dysmorphy-dystrophy. The other duct, cut across, shows clearer signs of cell necrobiosis: some nuclei are pale and hardly visible, others are flattened and hyperchromatic; finally, one intensely hematoxylinophilic cell shows a pycnotic nucleus and a swollen protoplasm that obstructs most of the lumen.

Before considering the characteristics of the parenchymal anomalies found in neonatal hepatitis, we will give a *brief indication of certain morphological images in relation with the histopathogenesis of neonatal hepatitis* which have been or are still a matter of discussion; as a result of the images proper and from their possible correlation or identification with those of viral hepatitis.

1. Problems Posed by the Images

a) SMETANA and JOHNSON [1955] do not find any eosinophilic bodies or necrosis of the cells followed by regeneration in neonatal hepatitis. However, EHRLICH and RATNER [1935] describe it in all stages of necrobiosis with eosinophilic staining of the protoplasm, vacuolization, nuclear picnosis and trabecular collapse.

b) According to SULZER and BROWN [1961] and CRAIG and LANDING [1952, chap. 2], in hepatitis with giant cells, the necrosis and complete destruction of the lobule is missing. However, DIBLE *et al.* [1954] observed a diffuse necrosis of the parenchymal cells in this type of hepatitis.

c) SMETANA and JOHNSON [1955] maintain that in neonatal hepatitis the 'ballooned' cells are not present; but CRAIG and LANDING [1952, chap. 2] have observed in all their cases a variation in the size of the cells and in the grade of their ballooning.

What interpretation could be given to these different morphopathological aspects pointed out by these authors? We underline the words of ATERMAN [1963], as it is not probable that the cited pathologists could disagree in the interpretation of simple pathological data or well-defined histopathological injuries, it should be accepted that neonatal hepatitis may produce a spectrum of alterations which do not have necessarily to be always present.

2. Histopathogenic Aspects in Relation to Viral Hepatitis

a) CRAIG and LANDING [1952, chap. 2] noted years ago the surprising histological similarity of the liver slides from children affected by neonatal hepatitis with those of biopsies from patients with viral hepatitis, whether epidemic or due to homologous serum.

To DIBLE *et al.* [1954] the lesions are essentially those of hepatitis or of diffuse hepatic cellular necrosis with the customary sequel of histocytic activity, fibrosis, ductal proliferation, and attempts at cellular regeneration.

b) To SMETANA and JOHNSON [1955], the histopathological changes observed in neonatal hepatitis are not very similar to the injuries observed in hepatitis at a later age.

EHRLICH and RATNER [1935] consider that the main objection to the acceptance of a viral cause (viral-hepatitic) in neonatal hepatitis is based on its histological characteristics. The fundamental changes in viral hepatitis should be present, as the limited development of the liver alters its response to the virus (serum hepatitis).

But, as ATERMAN [1963] has also pointed out, the main differences between these two apparently unrelated illnesses are the presence of degenerative changes and cellular necrosis in viral hepatitis, and the dominance of multinucleated cells in neonatal hepatitis.

The acute viral hepatitis in infancy, even when acquired in a very early period of extrauterine life, is histologically different from the image classified as 'neonatal hepatitis'. But it may be argued that such a difference is against the viral etiology of hepatitis with giant cells. Thus: (a) degenerative changes and cellular necrosis can also be found in hepatitis, as we have previously observed and as will be discussed later on, and (b) the presence of giant cells in neonatal hepatic-viral hepatitis corresponds to the expression in such a circumstance of the two types of situation in which such cells are present (p. 74).

B. Parenchymal Lesions

The parenchymal lesions evidenced by degeneration-necrobiosis and regeneration of the epithelial component in the hepatocyte and the epithelium of the excretory system in neonatal hepatitis is, in our experience, always visible although their extension and intensity are variable. Let us consider this in detail.

a) At the Hepatocyte Level

1. Degeneration-necrobiosis phenomena. According to CRAIG and LANDING [1952, chap. 2] these can be observed both in the nucleus, and the protoplasm.

a) In the nucleus: Loss of chromatin basophily, disappearance of nucleoli and eventually rupture of the nuclear membrane. In our series, these phenomena have also been prominent: hyperstaining of the chromatin, reduction of the nuclear size, and pyknosis.

b) In the protoplasm: Alteration of the reticular images and variable eosinophilia, sometimes with inclusion of materials of different nature (bile pigment, fat, etc., occasionally erythrocytes or leukocytes) (cpl. VIB).

2. Regenerative aspects. Usually, the cell appears enlarged, with one or several nuclei; multinucleated cells are larger in size. We are convinced that the multinucleated cells, which show their nuclei closely packed in a row or crowded together, are the product of nuclear division without division of the cytoplasm (syncytium), and are also regenerative elements; only the fact that these cells fail to individualize may indicate that they are degenerative elements, although it seems more logical to admit that they actually undergo a partial regeneration, which does not produce a complete hepatic cell. The giant cells with clearly separated nuclei, produced by union of protoplasms without union of nuclei (plasmodium),

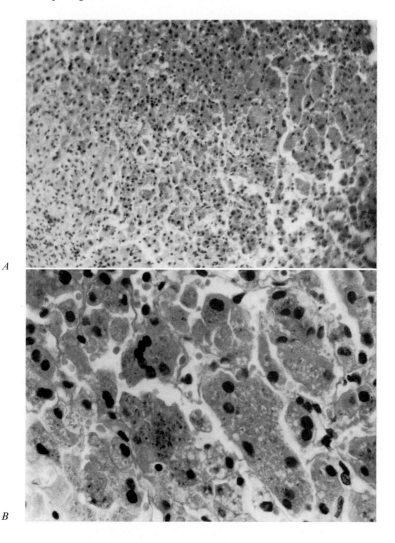

Fig. 9. A Case 8, as in colorplate VI. Left part of the image, a little more towards the right, to show the zone with more multinucleated cells. *B* Part of *A* at higher magnification. Two giant cells are clearly visible. One, towards the top and right of the image, is regenerative; another, towards the bottom and left, degenerative (for further detail, see p. 76).

may be interpreted, in our opinion, on the basis of the loss of cellular in-
dividuality, as clearly degenerative elements. From the disposition of the
nuclei it seems that certain giant cells correspond simultaneously to regenerative and degenerative phenomena in a given element. Moreover,
these cells can suffer a necrobiosis, as common hepatocytes do.

The regenerative aspect of the hepatocyte can also appear in the form of
polyploid nuclei. According to CRAIG and LANDING [1952, chap. 2], such elements
are not observed more frequently in the giant cells than in the normal ones. Again,
these cells with polyploid nuclei are vulnerable to necrobiotic agents.

b) At the Level of the Excretory System (Ducts)

Coetaneously with the process of alteration of the hepatocytes just
discussed, a process of deterioration or *degeneration-necrobiosis* takes
place in the ducts.

This process, that may be more obvious or less patent that the cellular anomalies, affects the ducts of the portal spaces, especially those of
Kiernan, and the ductules. More accurately, this process may be called
dysmorphy-dystrophy-necrobiosis – it is easily demonstrable on microscopic examination, although it has to be looked for to be proved. It leads
to lysis and disappearance of the structures and usually does not leave
any traces of its presence.

Beginning with a slight modification in the shape of the duct – which
could be dismissed as a result of an increased connective tissue pressure
due to an inflammatory reaction – to a total necrosis with a more or less
evident obliteration of the structure, it is possible to find a large number
of intermediate stages.

This d-d-n process of the excretory structures may be very clearly
observed in slides simply stained with the common hematoxylin and eosin
or trichromic methods. We believe that this process has not been considered with the attention it deserves. Only some authors, such as CRAIG and
LANDING [1952, chap. 2], have made some specific comments on it.
These authors pointed out the collapsed aspect of the ducts and the difficulty to distinguish them from the atresic ones; STOWENS [1966, chap. 2]
indicates that in the acute phase of the 'illness of the giant cells', the portal spaces appear compressed and the structures contained in them are often indistinguishable. This constitutes an important diagnostic point as
the impossibility to recognize the ducts makes one suspect that they are
absent. It is often impossible to determine, from a simple biopsy, the state
of the biliary system. In these cases, he recommends a second biopsy sev-

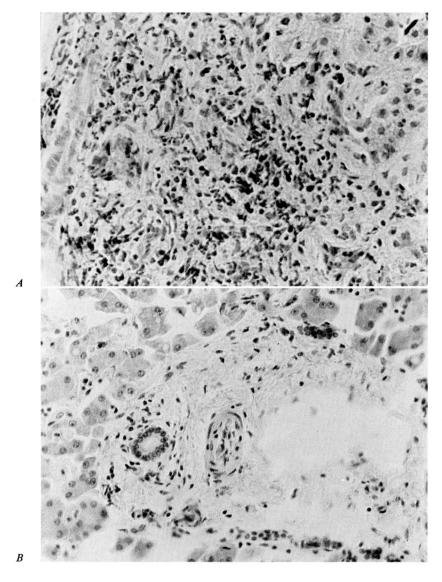

A

B

Cpl. VII. A Partial view of color plate I A at greater magnification. A septal duct is shown near a good-sized vessel which is dysmorphic, dystrophic, and with numerous devitalized nuclei: some of them are slightly colored; most of them are clearly pycnotic. This duct may be compared to a normal one shown in *B*. In the lower left of the picture another duct, obviously suffering the same process, may be seen. Some ductules and even some preductules appear damaged with similar lesions. *B* A normal portal duct, corresponding to the liver of an infant of the same age, who died from an acute respiratory process and with a moderate fatty hepatosis. Note two characteristic ductules at the top and bottom.

eral weeks later; at this time, if the ducts were present, they probably will
have become evident.

The collapsed, flattened aspect is usually the most apparent alteration of the ducts; but, in our opinion, the changes in the excretory structures (ducts and ductules) offer some features better defined by the mentioned trilogy. In section IV, we give our interpretation about the d-d-n
process which we believe is fundamental in the determinism of the inflammatory and atresia-inducing disease of the liver and bile ducts, and has
received so little attention[12].

Although the nomenclature of the pathological lesions is quite clear,
an account of their peculiar aspects must be presented.

1. Dysmorphy

Change in the configuration of the structure, which is normally
shown as follows:

a) Ducts

At the Structural Level

Wall: It shows a regular shape, channel-like in longitudinal sections,
and crown-like in transversal sections. In both cases, the wall is delineat-
ed by the cell nuclei, which are oval in shape and, in both types of section, they are set out vertically and parallel to each other.

Lumen: Clearly visible; usually it is roughly circular or oval in shape.

At the Cellular Level

The cells of the normal structure are cubic-prismatic, and the 'more
ductal' the structure the higher the cells are; in the septal ducts, they are
always clearly prismatic.

The dysmorphic structures, at the cellular level, show an abnormal
shape and, especially, an irregular disposition of the cells which appear
tilted and even flattened.

b) Ductules

These are very similar to the smaller ducts which are in continuity
with them: (1) with a smaller and often invisible lumen, and (2) with cubic or flattened cells with spheric or oval nuclei set out horizontally.

---

12   It has only been relatively recently [STRAUSS and BERNSTEIN, 1968] that the
degenerative alterations of the intrahepatic ducts have been considered in a more
definite way.

2. Dystrophy

a) In the channels: in a few cases larger, but usually smaller.

b) In the cells: rarely hypertrophic, but generally hypotrophic.

Dysmorphy and dystrophy, especially the former, are more manifest at the ductal than at the ductular level. A simple reason to account for this could be that the normal ductules already offer 'a certain aspect of dysmorphy-dystrophy' due to their structure, with a 'flattened disposition' of their cells.

3. Necrobiosis

Manifested by nuclear hyperpigmentation and pyknosis, karyorrhexis and karyolysis; sometimes the nuclei are hypochromatic, becoming very pale until they disappear. These nuclear changes are accompanied by degenerative alterations of the cytoplasm which is usually homogeneous, with variable eosinophilic hue, vacuolization, etc.

4. Lysis

This constitutes the final stage of the destructive process and obviously, does not show a typical appearance. Nevertheless, on occasion, an accumulation of connective inflammatory cells disposed in a circular pattern may be suggestive of the remains of a structure that has disappeared (fig. 6C).

The following figures show the d-d-n process affecting the excretory system in neonatal hepatitis: (a) in the type with abundant giant cell transformation (cpl. IA, VII); (b) in a case of neonatal hepatitis with a moderate number of giant cells (fig. 9B), and (c) in a case of hepatitis with very scarce giant cells (cpl. VIII).

C. Evolutive Prospects

The evolutive prospects of the d-d-n process may fall under the following patterns:

a) The d-d-n process, responsible of the real ductipenia, may show a continuous progressive increase, producing severe ductipenia or even a total obliteration and disappearance of ducts.

b) It may show a total regression of the lesions, a 'restitutio ad integrum' of the excretory structures. However, we believe that even when the organic reconstructive work is notorious, there is often a vestigial ductipenia, without affecting the functional capacity of the liver.

This has been confirmed in some of our cases controled by catamnestic studies. A good example of this situation could be our case 1 (p. 213), where the needle biopsy performed at the age of $8^1/_2$ years showed a clear shortage of ducts (although a percentile figure could not be given, as an insufficient number of portal spaces were obtained in the specimen). But such a relic has not produced any parenchymal defficiency up to date, when the boy is more that 12 years old. His serum alkaline phosphatase and lipid levels as well as his SGOP and SGPT values are within normal limits; he has only presented discreet mesenchymal analytic signs due to the hepatic fibrosis that have recently disappeared.

Finally, in relation with ductipenia (p. 51) some facts must be kept in mind:

In cases of severe portal cellular-edematous infiltration and in the absence of a necrosis-lysis, the ducts and ductules may become so *dysmorphic-dystrophic* that they are difficult to identify, or may even become completely unrecognizable with the histological staining techniques. In these cases there is no true ductipenia but a pseudoductipenia.

The histochemical techniques [phosphatases, leucinaminopeptidase, MORAGAS, 1968] may reveal such structures only when the functional impairment is slight or absent. Consequently, only a positive test of such enzymes will be of value to admit the existence of the structures, a negative test being of doubtful value, as it may correspond to a real absence of the structures or to a dysmorphy-dystrophy process with a lack of enzyme activity.

D. In neonatal hepatitis, at the same time as the d-d-n process affecting the excretory structures which we have just pointed out, a regeneration-proliferation phenomenon may be demonstrated as well. This will be discussed later on, when dealing with the dynamics of the injuries on page 88.

III. Intrahepatic Biliary Atresia

From a histopathogenic point of view, this entity may be considered essentially similar to the process causing extrahepatic atresia of the internal ducts, with a significant differential feature: the regeneration and hyperplasic phenomena are usually demonstrable, especially at the ductular level (cpl. XIB, XIIA), but of little intensity.

1. Considering which ducts have been affected and taking into account an eventual fibrous-cirrhotic proliferation, the following types of intrahepatic atresia can be noted [DANKS and CAMPBELL, 1966, chap. 2].

(a) atresia of the small ducts with persistence of the larger ones, either with or without cirrhosis; (b) atresia of the small ducts and of the larger ones, either with or without cirrhosis.

A careful and attentive observation of the excretory structure, preferably in a large specimen, will demonstrate a clear d-d-n process mainly in the ducts. Some authors [DANKS and CAMPBELL, 1966, chap. 2] refer to the necrosis of the ducts admitting a derangement of these structures. Therefore, these authors implicitly accept the existence of such a process, although they have not explicitly defined it. Recently, ALAGILLE et al. [1969, chap. 1] have pointed out that in intrahepatic atresia, the ducts of certain sections show an altered epithelium, with flattened cells, desquamating into the lumen, and with pycnotic nuclei. If serial sections are studied, the disappearance of the duct can be proved.

It is possible that some authors, when describing the hypoplasia of the ducts (p. 86), have been referring to the same process: if this is the case, the term they use is unfortunate as hypoplasia applies to a dysontogenic defect, whereas the actual process consists in the deterioration of adequately developed structures.

2. The histopathological image corresponding to intrahepatic atresia can often be observed in a very obvious and extensive fashion in mixed cases of intrahepatic and extrahepatic atresia, which are the most frequent type of atresias (p. 58). Some clear examples of this assertion (cpl. IX) follow.

We believe that this component of intrahepatic atresia in cases of extrahepatic atresia is practically constant: if carefully sought for in a large biopsy specimen, it is always possible to see it.

As KOOP [1968] points out, the longer the patient survives the more marked and extensive this component is. According to this author, the longer the course of the disease, the less ducts are found, and shortly before death practically none are left.

Opposing this concept of KOOP [1968], DANKS [1968] points out that a proliferative reaction of the ducts, with occasional segmental dilation, would exist in half the observations at the time of the child's death.

These opinions seem to be conflicting. However, we believe that it is only a problem of semantics. The ducts to which KOOP refers would be the ducts themselves, especially those of the septal spaces, while those noted by DANKS are the ducts of the small connective spaces and the ductules. Such interpretation would be in agreement with our own observations.

3. From a histopathogenic point of view, the isolated, pure form of intrahepatic biliary atresia is very similar or perhaps identical to the 'cho-

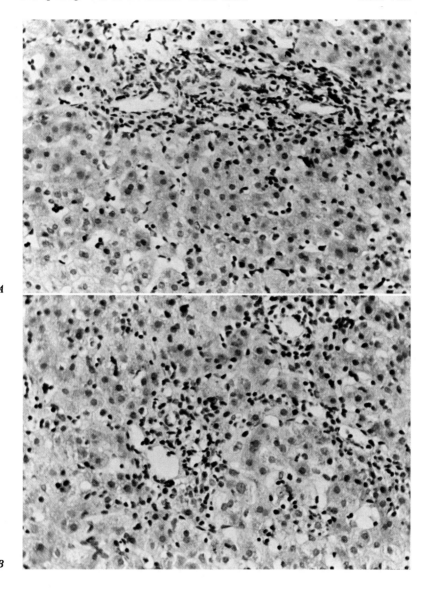

A

B

Cpl. VIII. Legend on reverse side of plate X.

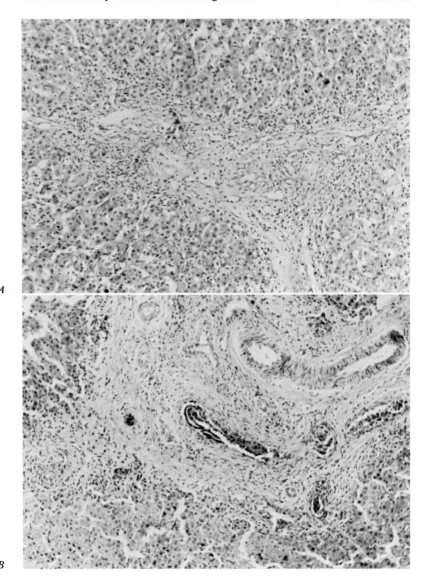

A

B

Cpl. IX. Legend on reverse side of plate X.

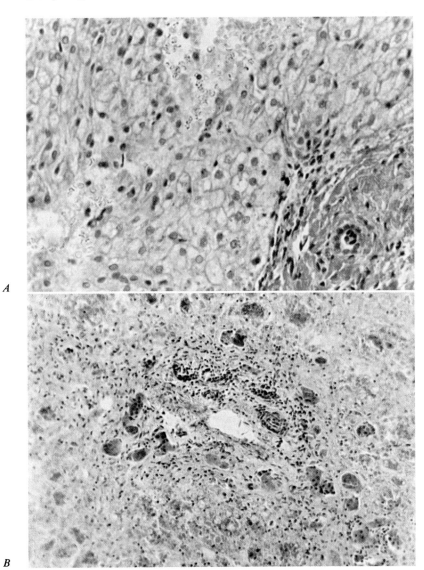

A

B

Cpl. X. Legend on reverse side.

The Inflammatory and Atresia-Inducing Disease

Legends for plate VIII–X

Cpl. VIII. A Needle biopsy of the liver corresponding to a neonatal jaundice producing hepatitis without total acholia but manifest at 2 ½ months of age. Biopsy performed at 3¹/₂ months of age (case 9, p. 222). Signs of intense portitis with an edematocellular infiltration and limited giant cell transformation. A good-sized portal space with several vessels is seen; its center shows a distorted duct, cut length ways. In the upper right part of the picture, a duct can be recognized, placed under the venule cut lengthways, between the hepatic trabecules. Another one above it runs parallel to the periphery of the lobule. Both show clear dysmorphy-dystrophy devitalization signs in their nuclei. *B* Three spaces of Kiernan. None of them has a duct. In the middle and top ones, nevertheless, there is a gathering of cells, probably corresponding to very distorted ductules. In another 6 connective spaces (apart from the 4 shown here), out of the 11 included in the needle biopsy specimen, the corresponding ductal structures were not visible either; only in one the duct appeared obviously normal. To sum up: was there real ductipenia (although unprovable) and/or nonrevealable pseudoductipenia or perhaps only a revealable pseudoductipenia? As the case could not be histochemically investigated there is no answer to these questions.

Cpl. IX. A Extrahepatic atresia, surgical biopsy performed at 2 months of age (case 10 p. 223). In this septum with light fibrosis and marked edema, furrowed by a good number of vessels and with sparse leukocytic infiltration, only a dysmorphic-dystrophic duct with mostly pycnotic elements is clearly visible. *B* Extrahepatic atresia. Surgical biopsy performed in a 55-day-old patient (case 4, p. 218). Septal fibrosis, with moderate ductal-ductular proliferation. In the center of the field, a great dysmorphic duct with clear signs of devitalization. Other ducts of smaller size are also severely deteriorated.

Cpl. X. A Neonatal hepatitis (as in cpl. VIII). Needle biopsy performed 5 months after clinical cure of the patient, although he still presented some abnormal laboratory findings (case 9, p. 222). Typical appearance of epithelial turnover in the duct of a small sept. *B* Acute atrophy following hepatitis, very probably of viral etiology, in a 3-month-old infant. Another case of the same nature occurred in the family. Extensive necrobiosis of the parenchyma with some preductules showing more lively appearance than the others.

langiolytic hepatitis', a denomination applied by BAGGENSTOSS [1966, chap. 2] to cases that reveal an *inflammatory destruction of the interlobular bile ducts* (the so-called cholangioles) or to a nonpurulent chronic destructive cholangitis clinically manifested by a syndrome of primary biliary cirrhosis. In studies on adults, this author finds that in such cholangiolytic hepatitis the number of interlobular ducts is significantly decreased to 0.38 per portal space; only in a few cases their number is normal, or increased to 1.4. Associated extra hepatic and intrahepatic atresia have an equivalent in the so-called 'sclerosing cholangitis' of the adult, a disease characterized by the progressive obstruction and obliteration of the extrahepatic bile ducts and later of the intrahepatic ones; WARREN *et al.* [HORTON, 1968] have recently published a series of observations on this disease.

4. The electron microscopic studies carried out by SHARP *et al.* [1967b, chap. 1] have revealed several anomalies of the canalicular structures. In some cases, the microvilli are projected into the canalicular lumen and seem to obstruct it; in others, the canaliculi are dilated and have lost their microvilli; even the cytoplasm can be seen projected into the lumen. Some canaliculi that contain accumulations of bile show nearly normal villi. The canaliculi with hypertrophy of the villi may be examples of a precocious duct formation [WOOD, 1966] or the result of a toxic action of the bile acids [SCHAFFNER and JAVIT, 1966]. As SHARP *et al.* [1967b, chap. 1] specifically point out, the interpretation of such electron microscopic findings should be viewed with caution, until more observations and more complete studies have been carried out.

5. The presence of inflammatory injuries with damage of the excretory structures proves the activity of the process. The decrease in the number of ducts (or its equivalent, the number of absent ones), the real evident ductipenia, offers decisive information about the extension of the atresia. A ductipenia without inflammatory signs should be interpreted as a very advanced phase of the process or perhaps as the final stage of the pathological course, when a complete atresia has practically been reached.

The pseudoductipenia, especially the revealable one, which results in a lesser functional impairment, has logically better possibilities of regeneration or reconstruction than the true ductipenia. When a true ductipenia reaches a great extension, a return to normality can hardly be expected; usually a functional disorder of varying severity will remain as an indelible manifestation (fig. 10).

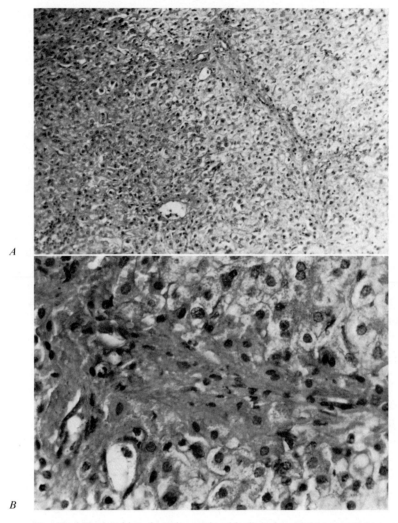

Fig. 10. A Neonatal intrahepatic atresia with clinical and laboratory data consistent with the diagnosis of a MacMahon-Thannhauser syndrome. Surgical biopsy at 3 years of age (case 14, p. 227). Portal spaces with hyalinized, fibrous connective tissue without any vestiges of ductal-ductular structures. *B* Partial view of *A* at greater magnification.

6. As has been mentioned on page 81, there is generally little ductular reaction in intrahepatic atresia. As is well known, a marked ductular proliferation is present: (a) In bile retention secondary to the blockade of the large ducts, and a similar result may be obtained following experi-

mental ligation of these ducts. (b) In noncholestasic acute viral hepatitis [DUBIN et al., 1960, chap. 1].

Similarly, a marked ductular proliferation in intrahepatic atresia might be expected. The fact that this proliferation is usually of small magnitude indicates, in our opinion, that the same agent causing the disease, a different cause, or perhaps an association of both, may inhibit to a greater or lesser degree such a proliferation.

IV. Why Attention Has Not Been Directed to the Process of Dysmorphy-Dystrophy-Necrobiosis, in All the Entities of the Triad, as Precursor of and Responsible for True Ductipenia

1. On occasion, there is only a dysmorphy-dystrophy or even a ductipenia, but not signs of ductal necrobiosis. In these cases, a banal cause, not damaging the duct, may be accepted. The cause, which is inferred, and which is accepted in an axiomatic fashion, is that the structure is only compressed, confused by the inflammatory exudation. Sometimes, this occurs with such an intensity that it gives the impression that the duct has disappeared, to reappear later once the exudate has been reabsorbed; i.e. that it was not a true ductipenia but only a pseudoductipenia. This might be too simple an explanation, acceptable only to a point. However, as a necrosis cannot be demonstrated, its existence may be doubted.

2. In cases with a complete d-d-n process, with evident necrobiosis. The necrobiosis to which we refer is not related, and cannot be mistaken, with the normal process of cellular turnover in the ducts, a constant feature in epithelial structures. In the physiological ductal cellular turnover, cells with varying degrees of necrobiotic changes are shed into the ductal lumen, but the remaining living cells offer a normal appearance, giving the duct an obvious eumorphism and eutrophia (cpl. X). Undoubtedly, to mistake a cellular shedding for a necrobiotic process grossly underrates the meaning of such a process.

a) A distinct appearance of necrobiosis, the event which really defines the d-d-n process in a complete fashion and gives it an outstanding value when it is demonstrated, is usually seen only in a few ducts: it is an unusual opportunity to observe it in many ducts at the same time. This applies not only to needle biopsy specimens, but also to the usual surgical biopsies. It is perhaps justifiable that the observation of necrobiotic phenomena, only in some isolated ducts, may be dismissed by the observer as something unimportant or not worth of attention. However, *nobody can deny, although it may be astonishing that a reduced number of laborers working during a certain time can build up a great work, even of gigantic proportions.*

b) Logically, the most common observation is the final result, i.e. ductipenia, rather than the ductal d-d-n process itself. This ductipenia gradually sets in during a relatively long time of evolution, and will remain obvious if there is no regenerative reaction, or only a modest one takes place. On the other hand, the necrobiosis does not even constitute a stage of the process, as it is a phenomenon that takes place in a relatively short time, and that will only be observed if the biopsy sample is obtained at the precise moment.

In summary: The number of ducts in necrobiosis as compared to that of the absent, or dysmorphic-dystrophic ones, may be so small that it is understandable that some authors might have overlooked them or have considered them to be unsignificant. In one of our cases of acquired Mac-Mahon-Thannhauser syndrome, for example, in which an extensive post-mortem study could be carried out, it was found that in 100 connective spaces there were 86 Kiernan spaces that showed:

Normal duct	0
Absent duct	70
Dysmorphic-dystrophic duct	10
Necrobiotic duct	6

and 14 septal spaces which revealed:

Normal ducts	7
Absent ducts	0
Dysmorphic-dystrophic duct or ducts	5
Necrobiotic duct or ducts	2

Conclusion: If the d-d-n process has been observed by some authors, it has been described above all with the confusing and inadequate term of hypoplasia.

Indeed, the structures can be of a smaller size, but we do not consider acceptable the term of hypoplasia, as this would connote a structure of subnormal dimensions due to diminished growth and is *commonly* understood, from a pathogenic point of view, as the result of an ontogenic defect which is responsible either of a scarce embryological development or a poor fetal growth, and from an etiological point of view, this would correspond to a genic disorder.

We believe that a more accurate term for this feature would be that of hypotrophy. With this, we imply a good embryonic development of the ducts which later on fail to grow, or even shrink as they decrease in size relatively or even absolutely, e.g. smaller weight, height and bulk of the organic structures in cases of marked hypotrophy or atrophy.

But certainly, the most descriptive and short term would be that of *dystrophy* as the microscopic study of these structures shows they are not reduced in size, but show also epithelial injuries witnessed by specific lessions: the process of d-d-n (p. 78).

Recently, LÜDERS [1974] has used the term hypoplasia in such a broad sense that he renders it both confusing and misleading. He even includes under such a term atresia itself; and not only when due to ontogenic trouble (developmental delay, malformation, etc.), but also when related to other causes (perhaps lack of use?, he wonders) acting on an originally normal biliary tract.

V. Dynamics of the Lesions in the Triad with Special Reference to the Regeneration-Proliferation and to the Dysmorphy-Dystrophy-Necrobiosis Process Suffered also by the Proliferated Cellular Elements

The lesions revealing the histopathogenesis of the entities of the triad are not, of course, static manifestations; on the contrary, they constitute the expression of a dynamic process which has a start, reaches a period of state, and follows an evolution, which may be: (1) towards a complete restoration; (2a) maintaining a continuous activity that will cause lesions of increasing severity in the organ itself and occasionally in other organs (the final point of the process may only be the death of the patient); (2b) in other cases the process heals, leaving more or less important sequelae, if there has been necrosis and destruction of tissues with production of a scar[13].

The concept that this is a dynamic process rather than a static one has already been referred to, especially in the case of extrahepatic atresia, in the works of KANOFF *et al.* [1953], GROSS [1953, chap. 1], REDO [1954], and CARLSON [1960]. Nevertheless, these authors refer to the dy-

13   With regard to the evolutive particularities of each of the entities of the triad, see chapter 9.

namics of these structures exclusively from an ontogenic point of view, as the manifestation of an embryological development which continues, they say, after birth. We think it is quite obvious that dynamics more than the mere development and growth of every structure towards acquiring the characteristics of adulthood is involved here. Properly, the embriological development has finished at the third to fourth month of intrauterine life. The process we witness is the result of an interrelation injury-reaction in the organism as a true *dynamic process*. The injury to a structure is accompanied by signs of activity to repair the injured areas.

According to our point of view, it seems easy to understand, for example: why neonatal hepatities sometimes courses to intrahepatic atresia [ANDERSEN and GHADIMI: cit. BENAVIDES *et al.*, 1942; VISAKORPI and SULAMAA, 1964; ALAGILLE, 1965; DANKS, 1968]; that extrahepatic atresia can offer signs of regeneration of its injured ducts, with the possibility of becoming surgically amenable after having been previously inoperable or, even, of achieving spontaneous repermeabilization in infrequent cases; that a case of atresia successfully operated, performing an anastomosis, may be followed by the disappearance of the pathological-clinical signs of secondary fibrosis (cirrhosis) which existed before the intervention [cases of CAMERON and BUNTON, 1960, chap. 1; THALER and GELLIS, 1968a–d, chap. 1; KASSAI *et al.*, 1968, chap. 1].

1. The dynamics of the process are clearly exposed when considering the microscopic demonstration of signs of destruction and reaction of the organism; the latter ones consisting in the regeneration-proliferation phenomena which may be demonstrated in all the entities.

The regeneration-proliferation of the glandular parenchymal element, of the hepatocyte, has already been referred to (p. 76) and we dealt with such a phenomenon when discussing the alterations of the excretory structures (pp. 66, 78 and 82) in the sections on histopathogenesis of the entities of the triad. Let us now elaborate further into the dynamics of this injury-reaction process, determined by a regeneration-proliferation at the bile duct level, because it has a high speculative value when considering the pathogeny of the triad.

HANAI *et al.* [1967, chap. 2] have studied the morphology of the proliferated bile ducts in atresia and related hepatic illnesses using the tridimensional study technique.

Briefly explained, the images observed by these authors are as follows:

a) Extrahepatic atresia: The portal space contains all the elements: artery, vein, lymphatic vessels, the duct, and a mass of proliferated ductules which may be mistaken for the duct by its size, lumen, and course. In contrast to intrahepatic atresia, the ductules are not blind-ended. A great distorsion of the proliferated ductules is evident, with irregularities in their shape, size, and disposition; cellular damage is evident. The great distorsion of such excretory structures makes it difficult to distinguish ductules from tubular-shaped hepatic trabecules. There are bile thrombi within the proliferated ductules.

b) Intrahepatic atresia: In this type, there are no ducts in the portal spaces; nevertheless, if extensive portions of the gland are studied, remnants of such structures may be found in some areas. Besides, two kinds of portal spaces are demonstrated: one with a badly distorted and blindended duct, foating in the connective tissue, and another without a duct and with some ductular proliferation, consisting of dilated ductules near the union with the parenchyma, which become narrow to end blindly, and without bile content.

c) Hepatitis: The limitant plate is interrupted at various points, presenting a saw-like aspect. The interlobular duct is abnormal. In some areas, it thins out and disappears; in others, it shows a moderate proliferation. The ductules also show areas of proliferation, but not as profusely as in extrahepatic atresia. Thrombi of inspissated bile are found in some ducts and ductules.

Two points mentioned by these authors when considering intrahepatic atresia should be pointed out: (1) the authors do not dare predict if such ducts and ductules are on their way to disappear or to proliferate and extend, and (2) they do admit that cirrhosis apparently has not reached an advanced enough stage of development to cause the disappearance of ducts and ductules.

Applying our own observations to these specific points, we would advance the following comments: (1) The process is a mixed case of destruction and proliferation; in the particular case of intrahepatic atresia, the former predominates. (2) Both in intrahepatic and extrahepatic atresias, and in hepatitis, as well, interstitial fibrosis does not appear to be the main cause of deterioration of such a structures; some other cause or agent must be responsible for such changes.

2. The process of regeneration-proliferation has, to us, a high speculative value, considered from a pathogenic point of view, due to the following basic reasons:

a) Because of the special circumstance of *being observable with varying intensity in the three entities,* as we already indicated.

It cannot accurately be defined to which extent preductules, ductules, and ducts, respectively, participate in this process of regeneration-proliferation which may be found in each of the entities of the triad, but most prominently in extrahepatic atresia without intrahepatic component.

However, the following facts about this process can be established:

Specifically referring to extrahepatic atresia, some authors, e.g. ALAGILLE *et al.* [1969], maintain that such regeneration-proliferation process is of 'neo-canalicules' (perilobular ducts, i.e. ductules). Other authors, e.g. DANKS and CAMPBELL [1966, chap. 2] consider that the regeneration-proliferation process takes place at ductal level.

The predominant location of the process, in a juxtaparenchymal situation, suggests that the ductules are those with a more predominant participation.

The ductules, as a less differentiated structure than the ducts, should have greater regenerative capabilities. The ductal epithelium offers a mature, prismatic configuration; the preductules, on the other hand, have partly acquired the characteristics of the hepatocytes, cells with a larger protoplasm, and their regenerative capacity should be less than that of the ductules.

According to our thesis, dedifferentiation of the ducts takes place prior to or simultaneously with proliferation, with the prismatic epithelium of the ducts becoming cuboidal; color plate XIVA is, we believe, very demonstrative to this respect. The proliferation, even when papillary in type, exhibits a cuboidal epithelium or a flat one in some areas. We believe it is beyond any doubt that these are proliferated ducts; because such structures appear surrounded by a wide connective band that separates them considerably from the lobule; this situation clearly corresponds to that of a duct.

With regard to the proliferation of the preductules, which on occasion is quite obvious (cpl. IVB), it is difficult to state whether there is a true proliferation or only a transformation of the hepatic trabecules into preductules. Actually, a certain degree of tubular transformation is found in cholestasis; it can even be demonstrated in the innermost portion of the lobule, near the central lobular vein. These tubular structures show, at the light microscope, a morphology practically identical to the preductular ones. As, on the other hand, these preductules show no signs of mitotic divisions, the existence of either a true proliferation, or of only a transformation, or of both processes at a time, cannot be easily asserted. We believe however, that the preductules also take part in such a regeneration-proliferation. If the preductules are capable of proliferating in hepatic atrophy (cpl. XB), a similar response may be expected to occur in the entities of the triad, and probably even with more intensity in extrahepatic atresia with no component of intrahepatic atresia.

b) To us the process of regeneration-proliferation assumes a great significance in the determinism of the entities of the triad due to the fact that *in such regenerated-proliferated structures the d-d-n process may appear,* as it usually does, with varying intensity.

In the literature, no clear reference to this contingency of the regenerated-proliferated structures has been found: e.g. both in the first edition (p. 506) and in the second (p. 616) of *Pediatric Pathology* by STOWENS, there is a picture with proliferated ducts in a case of congenital biliary atresia in which a d-d-n is quite manifest, and yet, it is not mentioned in the text; it is simply stated that in atresia, the proliferated ducts are always abnormal, with an irregular epithelium or of an embryonic type.

In recent papers by BROUGH and BERNSTEIN [1969, chap. 1] and by ALAGILLE *et al.* [1969, chap. 1; 1969], no direct mention is made of the d-d-n process that can be suffered by the proliferated excretory structures. Somewhat more explicit are HANAI *et al.* [1967, chap. 2] who, when considering the irregularities in shape and size of the proliferated ductules, cite incidentally the cellular damage, without discussing it any further.

3. Some microphotographs provide the demonstration of this process of regeneration-proliferation and of its possible contingency, d-d-n; this is a total process that can be classified as *proliferation-degeneration*.

a) The proliferation-degeneration is mainly seen in extrahepatic atresia. The case shown in color plate XIA is a good example.

b) A process of proliferation-degeneration is also evident, although with less intensity, in intrahepatic biliary atresia. A very demonstrative case is depicted in color plates XIB and XIIA.

c) Finally, concerning the proliferation-degeneration process in *neonatal hepatitis,* it may be briefly and schematically said that it usually acquires an intermediate degree between both atresisa: pure extrahepatic (without any component of intrahepatic atresia) and intrahepatic.

Attention must be drawn to color plates IA and VIIA, where apart from two perfectly visible d-d-n ducts, ill-defined neoducts and neoductules can be seen among the inflammatory magma, showing an abnormal image.

In color plate VIA, corresponding to a neonatal hepatitis with a small number of giant cells, the upper part of the connective space exhibits a d-d-n duct, containing bile and the lower at higher magnification (cpl. XIIB) another good example of proliferation-degeneration.

VI. Other Histopathological and Histopathogenetic Aspects of the Inflammatory and Atresia-Inducing Process

A. Histopathological Aspects

The *inflammatory infiltrates* contain mononucleated leukocytes, neutrophiles and, sometimes, a fair number of eosinophils; usually there are only a few plasma cells. The neutrophiles are sometimes particularly abundant in acute processes, but not as much as is usually seen in ascending cholangitis due to intermittent obstruction of the external bile ducts, e.g. in the case of a common bile duct cyst.

Given the scarcity of plasma cells and the fact that *the necrobiosis of the hepatocytes usually has an irregular distribution,* a 'piecemeal necrosis' pattern does not result, thus suggesting that autoagressive mechanisms do not play a significant role or at least, that they act in a nonspecific fashion. Furthermore, the investigation of autoantibodies (tissue antibodies: nuclear and others) in congenital atresia is negative [DONIACH and WALKER, 1969].

B. Histopathogenetic Aspects
1. Significance of the Inflammatory Signs that Are Usually Included in the Pathological Background of Atresia

The inflammatory cellular infiltration generally present in atresia is, like that in hepatitis, thought to be consubstantial with the etiological primary cause of the disorder; however, it may be, in fact, secondary to bile stasis.

It is a well-known fact [recently confirmed by HESS, 1961, chap. 2] that bile stasis can produce inflammatory lesions and organic-functional disorders in the supra-obstructive structures; ducts and parenchyma are especially affected in cases of partial obstruction, probably due to an associated infective component.

The difficulties to even distinguish between external obstructive, occlusive, and parenchymal jaundice have once more been pointed out by SOTGIU [1965], who studied the lesions of the biliary tract in hepatitis. By systematic studies of the sediment as well as by chemical and electrophoretic analysis of the bile collected by duodenal aspiration, coupled with duodenal biopsies, this author found that the large bile ducts and the duodenal mucosa are frequently altered in acute hepatitis, and that this alteration in certain cases contributes to the persistence of jaundice. Thus, SOTGIU [1965] divides hepatitis into an exclusively hepatic type and a hepatoangiobiliary one. PAVEL and PIEPTEA [1966] have reached similar conclusions in their work. These findings revive, to a certain extent, the very classic concept of the 'mucous plug' of VIRCHOW.

The production of inflammatory phenomena occurs even in the experimental ligation of the bile ducts, as was already indicated (p. 73). Finally, according to the electron microscopy studies by HOLLANDER and SCHAFFNER [1968, chap. 1], the cellular changes in the hepatocyte, induced by simple obstruction by ligation of the ducts, are not distinguishable from those seen in viral hepatitis.

From what has been said, biliary stasis may reasonably be considered as the cause of inflammation, as the following diagram indicates.

$$\text{Hepatopathy} \rightarrow \left\{ \begin{array}{ll} \text{Inflammatory action} & \rightleftarrows \\ \text{destructive action} & \rightleftarrows \\ \text{excretory deficiency} & \rightleftarrows \end{array} \right\} \text{Cholestasis}$$

The destructive action causes atresia of the ducts and ductules. The excretory deficiency, cellular and canalicular, may be due to a thickening of the bile or to some other cause.

But without an obvious obstructive cause, neither extrinsical nor intrinsical, how can the production of atresia be explained? As will be seen later (chap. 6. VII), it takes place in the majority of cases in the late fetal or neonatal period, when the liver has already shown clear signs of functional activity, with signs of patency of the biliary tract (normal meconium).

The existence of a *primary* process causing the destruction of the epithelium will have to be admitted; this destruction will be followed by a connective tissue proliferation giving rise to a scar which fills the lumen and causes the atresia. And *this argument is*, we believe, *unquestionable* in the case of *cholestasis due to total atresia*, extrahepatic and intrahepatic, in which any ductular proliferation hardly exists or is even missing (example, case 10, p. 223, cpl. IXA).

Should the inflammatory reaction be of a secondary type, there would be no reason to expect a decrease in the inflammatory process; on the contrary, it would have to increase as the atresia remained unmodified. What actually occurs is that the inflammatory component shows a tendency to decrease, to recede clearly as the process continues.

Many authors have had the opportunity to determine the decrease of the inflammatory infiltration in the evolutive course of the hepatopathy; we have also confirmed it in some of our observations. With PILLOUD [1966, chap. 1], we believe that if inflammatory signs are not found at the time of the histological observation, it is because these have already receded, the injury having reached the resolution or scarring phase with sequelae.

2. Atrophy of the Epithelium

Recently, NEGRO and LARGUERO [1965], in agreement with preceding authors, pointed out that atresia does not result from atrophy of the epithelium, but is due to pathological processes originated in the connective tissue. DANKS *et al.* [1968, chap. 2] also refer to the progressive sclerosis of the ducts inside the liver and classify their reduction in size and number as hypoplasia.

Two aspects of this problem are worth discussion:

1. We think that the term 'ductal hypoplasia' is inadequate, as frequent signs of cellular proliferation can be observed both in normal cells and in cells wtih necrobiotic changes, as may be seen in color plate XIII.

As previously mentioned (pp. 67, 87), we think it is more accurate to refer to hypotrophy or, better, dystrophy, so that it does not imply a developmental defect, but a series of biological changes caused mainly by an interference with the complex nutritional-reproductive functions at the cellular level.

2. It should be pointed out that according to our observations, lesions of the connective tissue or a mere sclerosis can only occasionally be held responsible for the d-d-n process, as they could somehow suffocate the excretory epithelial structures. Although the possibility of this contingency, due to the mesenchymal involvement, seems to us undeniable, we believe that the agent which is causing the inflammation is, at least to a good extent, directly responsible for the dysmorphy and especially for the dystrophy and necrobiotic process.

The reasons on which we base our assertion are: (a) Some cases with severe lesions of inflammatory infiltration show only moderate or slight alterations of the epithelial elements. (b) Very often, there is edema of the fibrous tissue; the metabolic exchanges of the epithelial lining in these cases should not be seriously endangered (cpl. IXA). (c) On occasion, the d-d-n component is very apparent and extensive, whereas the infiltrative and fibrous mesenchymal reaction is slight or practically absent.

3. Papillary Proliferation
In some cases, even with marked fibrous proliferation and varying leukocytic infiltration, a great ductule-ductal proliferation and even a marked *ductal proliferation of a papillary type* may be seen (cpl. XIVA); there is an incresae not only in the number of thes structures but also in their size.

4. Vitality of the Structures
In some processes with great connective proliferation, as in congenital hepatic fibrosis and fibroangiomatosis of the bile ducts, a proliferation of the bile ducts in the midst of a markedly fibrotic tissue may be seen; this would be a proof that *the vitality of the structures is not exclusively connective-dependent* (cpl. XIVB).

5. Fibrosis-Cirrhosis
In all the entities of the triad, as an expression of the vascular-connective reaction appearing in all inflmamatory processes with the purpose of replacing the destroyed structures, and as a manifestation of symbiosis with the ductal-ductal proliferation in response to the bile retention, a

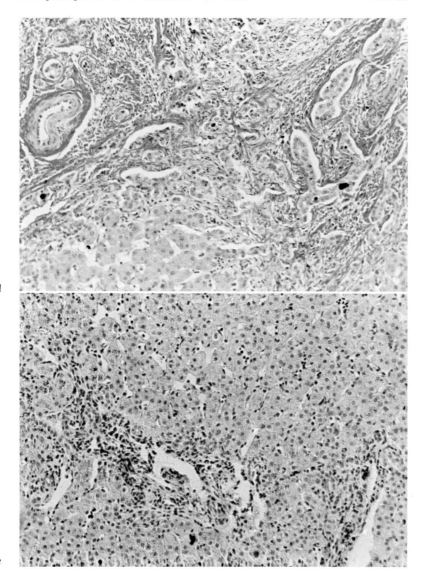

A

B

Cpl. XI. Legend on reverse side.

Legend for plate XI

Cpl. XI. A Case 2 (p. 215). Liver specimen. Autopsy performed at 4 months and 11 days of age in a patient, with extrahepatic atresia. Crown of neoductules and neoducts around a lobule, in which the furthest ones show a clear dysmorphy-dystrophy and in some others even total necrobiosis. Note that the intensity of the d-d-n process is not parallel to the fibrous proliferation. The newly formed structures show less vitality where the connective tissue is most lax (top part of the image). *B* A case of neonatal intrahepatic atresia, preferentially affecting the ducts of the small septa, later classified as a complete clinical and analytical MacMahon-Thannhauser syndrome. Liver biopsy obtained in the surgical exploration practiced at 7 weeks of age (case 11, p. 223). A careful scanning of the slide will show some images like the one shown here: small septum with notorious leukocytic infiltration and in which the normal ducts are not visible; in one of its corners a marked proliferation of ducts leave the lobule or contact intimately with the limiting plates; at most, a single connective cellular layer separates them; hence nearly all of them are ductules offering a paranormal aspect, with clear dysmorphy-dystrophy. A view at a larger magnification proves these statements (cpl. XII A).

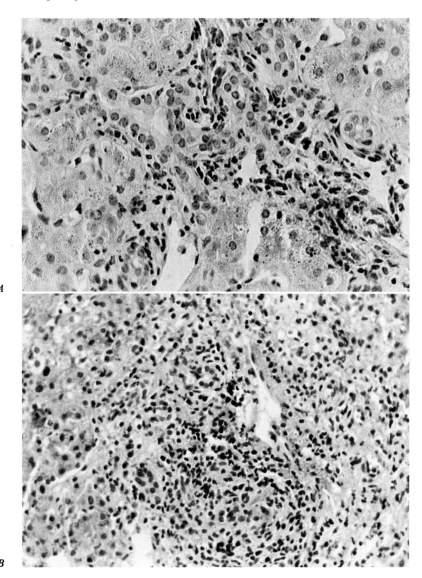

A

B

Cpl. XII. Legend on reverse side.

Legend for plate XII

Cpl. XII. A A detail at higher magnification of a corner of the septum from color plate XI B. *B* Neonatal hepatitis. Surgical biopsy (case 8, p. 221). Lower part of color plate VI A. Five ducts can be recognized, more than would correspond to this space, indicating a regeneration-proliferation process. The uppermost duct is practically normal, with only some pycnotic nuclei, but with a well-outlined lumen. The other 4 ducts are clearly dysmorphic-dystrophic, especially the lowest one which is cut lengthways. One can suspect the presence of ducts and even of some ductules, but so modified that their presence cannot be demonstrated.

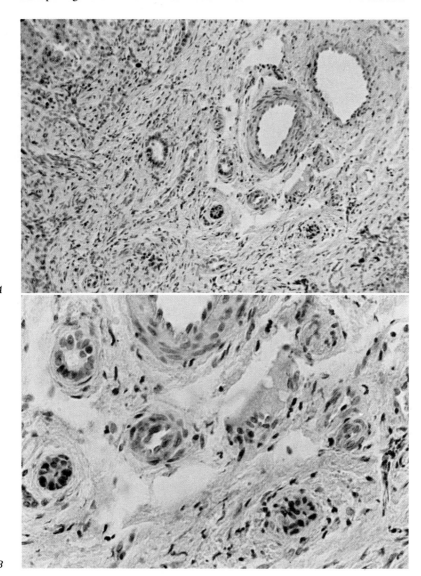

A

B

Cpl. XIII. Legend on reverse side.

The Inflammatory and Atresia-Inducing Disease

Legend for plate XIII

Cpl. XIII. A Atresia of the great intrahepatic ducts near the hilum. Surgical biopsy (case 7, p. 220). Septal space of great size with large vessels and a nerve; the space shows marked fibrous perilobular ductular-ductal proliferation. Outside the proliferative band, within the connective tissue of the septum, 6 ducts with various degrees of vitality may be seen. *B* Detail of *A* at higher magnification, which includes 3 of the 6 ducts. Two of them, to the right of the picture, surrounded by connective tissue with equal cellular-fibrillar characteristics, and show a different degree of vitality; the lower one is clearly necrobiotic. Some nuclei arranged in 2 levels, indicate a certain amount of proliferation.

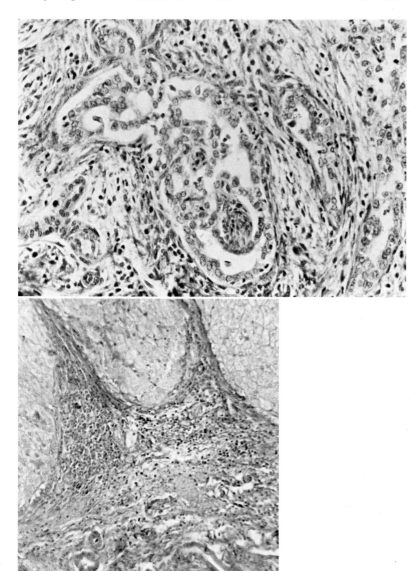

A

B

Cpl. XIV. Legend on reverse side.

The Inflammatory and Atresia-Inducing Disease

Legend for plate XIV

Cpl. XIV. A Case 4 (p. 218). Surgical biopsy of the liver performed in the 55th day of life in a baby with extrahepatic atresia. Very marked septal fibrosis, with patent leuko-cytic infiltration, in spite of the short time of extrauterine life. The ductal proliferation is manifest in the formation of discrete but quite obvious papillary structures. Comparison with color plate VII B unquestionably proves how the ductal epithelium even with an adenomatous shape is lower, more cuboidal, or flatter, than that in the normal ducts. *B* Congenital hepatic fibrosis with moderate angiomatous changes in the bile ducts. Septum with marked fibrosis, causing a remarkable roundness of the lobules; many ducts with a prismatic epithelium, which is moderately high and only slightly hypotrophic, are present [case observed by SORIANO *et al.*].

more or less active and extensive fibrous proliferation may be found. When such a proliferation is accompanied by an obvious functional disorder of the parenchyma, it will be labeled as a cirrhosis.

These are the most relevant features of this fibrosis-cirrhosis:

1. Its evolution does not show a time-related pattern. Sometimes, in a short time of evolution, an intense fibrosis has already developed (cpl. XIVA); on occasion, the process of connective hyperplasia is low. Nevertheless, the fibrocirrhotic process in extrahepatic atresia, the entity where it can be more easily seen, appears, as a rule, after the sixth week of extrauterine life. We believe this to mean that even in such a type of atresia, the most 'obstructive' of all the entities of the triad, the onset of cholestasis does not take place during intrauterine life. Two reasons may explain this: (1) little bilirubin is elaborated by the fetal liver, and (2) the unmodified bilirubin is eliminated via the placenta. The intense cholestasis and the fibrous-cirrhotic reaction begin to develop after birth, from the moment the blockage to bile excretion occurs and becomes ostensible after a period of time.

2. The fibrosis-cirrhosis does not constitute an irreversible process; even an intense fibrosis due to extrahepatic atresia can recede after surgical reestablishment of the bile flow [cases of CAMERON and BUNTON, 1960, chap. 1; THALER and GELLIS, 1968a–d, chap. 1; KASSAI *et al.*, 1968, chap. 1]. There is experimental evidence to prove that a cirrhotic liver can recover; hence, cirrhosis is not an irreversible process. BELL [1926], CAMERON and OAKLEY [1932] in dogs and cats, and more recently CAMERON and PRASAD [1960] in rats, have demonstrated that a severe biliary cirrhosis secondary to the ligation of the common bile duct can disappear completely. This is achieved by proliferation of the liver cells, dedifferentiation of the intrahepatic bile ducts and formation of many new lobules. The fibrous tissue is partially incorporated into the framework of the regenerating lobules and part of it disappears. Nevertheless, a limit to the regenerating capacity of the liver does exist; beyond that the liver cannot recover.

3. In extrahepatic biliary atresia the process tends to adopt the aspect of the classical secondary biliary cirrhosis, due to external cholestasis.

4. In neonatal hepatitis, the fibrocirrhotic process tends to be ill-defined.

5. A similar appearance is usually found in intrahepatic atresia, although occasionally it can show the aspect of primary biliary cirrhosis. We have observed this in one of our patients with an acquired MacMahon-Thannhauser syndrome, whose jaundice began when the infant was $4^1/_2$ months old.

VII. Histopathogenic Synthesis

Especially in the portal spaces of Kiernan, an important event takes place: the development of an inflammatory process with deleterious characteristics which can be classified according to the state of the excretory structures.

1. A dysmorphy-dystrophy-necrobiosis process affects mostly the ducts, and the dynamics of their reaction to injury offer signs of regeneration-proliferation concerning usually the ductules.

2. When there is a marked vascular-exudative component, ducts and ductules become indistinct, being sometimes *impossible* to distinguish them among the infiltrative elements. As a result, the d-d-n process or the regeneration-proliferation phenomenon which may be taking place in them cannot be evidenced in its real extent.

That is why it is possible to refer to *ductipenia* (or perhaps ductulipenia) which may be real and/or fictitious (pseudoductipenia). The *real* one corresponds to a complete d-d-n process which led to death and disappearance of the structures; the *pseudoductipenia*, corresponds to an incomplete d-d-n process; there is only dysmorphy and dystrophy, but to such a degree that the lumen of the structures becomes a virtual space, unidentifiable under the microscope; perhaps histochemical methods could reveal them.

We emphasize that the pseudoductipenia corresponds mainly to the smallest ducts, in the portal spaces of Kiernan, and not so frequently to those in the larger portal spaces, the septal ones, where the ducts display their well-defined and unmistakable histological structure: a high prismatic epithelium and an adventitial layer of varying thickness and circumferential collagen bundles, clearly different from the rest of the connective tissue.

3. The histopathogenic characteristics of the entities of the triad indicate quite clearly that they *merely evidence the existence* of a *hepatic inflammatory process* with an obvious and more or less extensive *dystrophying-necrosizing character* in the excretory system. This process has not been clearly identified and described so far and yet it is the key to explain both extrahepatic and intrahepatic atresia. This *process of dystrophy and necrobiosis is accompanied by a regeneraiton of the structures*, or even by hyperplasia. Usually regeneration fails to take place when affecting the large ducts, ending with the replacement of the injured structures by a connective scar tissue. As to the possible recovery of the damaged structures in both types of ductipenia, pseudoductipenia has logically a much better prognosis, whereas in true ductipenia, especially when involving the septal ducts, a poor outcome must be expected.

4. When atresia is not very extensive and the bile flow can be artifically restored, the process can subside to a point where a normal function of the liver may be achieved.

5. The atresia-inducing inflammatory process usually begins *in utero* and progresses throughout the initial period of extrauterine life; with marked atresia of the excretory ducts, only rarely may be seen beyond 3 months of age. In effect:

a) *Isolated* extrahepatic atresia can be compared pathogenically only with stenosis of the main bile duct, not etiologically due to surgical aggression or traumatism and which is not associated to other pathogenical elements (calculosis, injuries of the duodenum and pancreas, etc.) which determine the obliteration. Such a disease is infrequent in the adult, according to the data of LAHEY and PYRTEK [1950], ARANDES *et al.* [1963], etc., and even more in pediatric pathology.

b) Extrahepatic atresia *associated to the intrahepatic type* can be compared pathogenically with 'sclerosing cholangitis' of the adult (p. 83) a disease which is not common either.

c) *Pure* intrahepatic atresia can be compared at least in some aspects to 'cholangiolithic hepatitis' with or without an associated syndrome of primary biliary cirrhosis, in which – according to BAGGENSTOSS [1966, chap. 2] – the ductipenia tends to be pronounced (p. 83).

This neonatal intrahepatic atresia could be identified with a process appearing in later age, after the first 3 months, which could be labeled as 'acquired MacMahon-Thannhauser syndrome', with jaundice appearing after the mentioned date as its most outstanding sign.

Few observations of this syndrome have been reported so far. Our data, probably incomplete, include: a case from JOSEPH *et al.* [1959] in a child of 1½ years; another of ALAGILLE *et al.* [1962] in a child of 5 years; another in a moman of 46 years [BLATRIX *et al.,* 1963]; two observations of our own in collaboration with A. LLORENS TEROL in two siblings from a consanguineous couple. Recently, ALAGILLE *et al.* [1969, chap. 1] have reported other cases within their series of 25 patients with intrahepatic biliary atresia and patent external bile ducts which they classify as follows: 14 out of 25 (56%) of neonatal origin; 1 which started at the age of 5 months; 8 (32%) in childhood, and 2 which began at an undetermined age.

References

ALAGILLE, D.; COCHARD, A. M. et LE TAN VINH: Absence congénitale de voies biliaires intrahépatiques. Revue méd. fr. *37:* 57 (1962).

ALAGILLE, D.; GAUTIER, M.; HABIB, E. C. et DOMMERGES, P.: Les donnés de la biopsie hépatique pre- et per-opératoire au cours des cholestases prolongées du nourrisson. Archs fr. Pédiat. *26:* 297 (1969).

ANDERSEN, D. H.: cit. BENAVIDES *et al.* (chap. 1).

ARANDES, R.; BALLESTER, J. y. ALCALDE, R. P.: in Afecciones de la vía biliar principal (Ed. JIMS, Barcelona 1963).

ATERMAN, K.: Neonatal hepatitis and its relation to viral hepatitis of the mother. Am. J. Dis. Child. *105:* 395 (1963).

BELL, L. P.: cit. CAMERON and BUNTON (chap. 1).

BLATRIX, C.; LANCRET, P.; GERMAIN, A. et GREGOIRE, D.: La cholostase chronique de l'adulte. A propos d'un cas de maladie de MacMahon-Thannhauser. Presse méd. *71:* 230 (1963).

CAMERON, R. and OAKLEY, L.: cit. CAMERON and BUNTON (chap. 1).

CAMERON, R. and PRASAD, L. B. M.: cit. CAMERON and BUNTON (chap. 1).

CARLSON, E.: Salvage of the 'noncorrectable' case of congenital extrahepatic biliary atresia. Archs Surg., Chicago *81:* 893 (1960).

DANKS, D. M.: Answer to the letter of the editor (E. Koop). J. pediat. Surg. *3:* 592 (1968).

DIBLE, J. H.; JUNT, W. E.; PUGH, V. M.; STEINGOLD, L., and WOOD, J. H. F.: Foetal and neonatal hepatitis and its sequelae. J. Path. Bact. *67:* 195 (1954); cit. ATERMAN.

DONIACH, D. and WALKER, J. G.: A unified concept of autoimmune hepatitis. Lancet *i:* 813 (1969).

EHRLICH, J. C. and RATNER, I .M.: Congenital cirrhosis of the liver with kernikterus. Report of two cases in siblings with a discussion of the relationship to so-called neonatal hepatitis and to isoimmunization disease. Am. J. Path. *31:* 1013 (1935); cit. ATERMAN.

ESTERLY, J. R.; SLUSSER, R. J., and RUEBNER, B. H.: Hepatic lesions in the congenital rubella syndrome. J. Pediat. *71:* 676 (1967).

GHADIMI, H.: cit. BENAVIDES *et al.* (chap. 1).

GREWE, H. E.: Zur operativen Behandlung der Gallengangsatresie. Zentbl. Chir. *89:* 145 (1964).

JOSEPH, R.; NEZELOFF, C.; RIBIERRE, M. et JOB, J. C.: Ictère cholostatique chronique par angiolite et péricholangiolite (syndrome de MacMahon) chez un enfant de 18 mois. Sem. Hôp. Ann. Péd. *35:* 2123, P/337 (1959).

KANOF, A.; DONORAN, E., and BERNER, H.: Congenital atresia of the biliary system. Delayed development of correctability. Am. J. Dis. Child. *86:* 750 (1953).

KOOP, E.: Commentary ot the pargaraph of DANKS *et al.* J. pediat. Surg. *3:* 592 (1968).

LAHEY, F. and PYRTEK, L. S.: Experience with operative management of 280 structires of the bile ducts with description of a new method and complete followup study of end results in 229 of the cases. Surgery Gynec. Obstet. *91:* 25 (1950).

LÜDERS, D.: Hypoplasie der intrahepatischen Gallengänge und andere Formen intrahepatischen Cholestase im Säuglingsalter. Mschr. Kinderheilk. *122:* 207 (1974).

MORAGAS, A.: Histochemical diagnosis of biliary atresia. Lancet *ii:* 556 (1968).

NEGRO, R. C. y LARGUERO, P. I.: in NEGRO, GENTILE RAMOS y RAMÓN GUERRA Enfermedades del hígado en la infancia (Delta Panamerica, Buenos Aires 1965).

Pavel, I. und Pieptea, R.: Die Rolle des Duodenums in protahierten oder rezidivie-
renden Hepatitisfällen. Münch. med. Wschr. *108:* 26 (1966).

Reo, S. F.: Congenital atresia of the extrahepatic bile ducts. Archs Surg., Chicago
69: 886 (1954).

Rickham, P. P.: Neonatal jaundice surgical aspects. Clin. Pediat. *3:* 197 (1964).

Schaffner, F. N. and Javitt, B.: Morphologic changes in hamster liver during
cholestasis induced by taurolithocolate. Lab. Invest. *15:* 1783 (1966).

Singer, D. B.; Rudlph, A. J.; Rosenberg, H. S.; Rawls, W. E., and Boniuk, M.:
Pathology of the congenital rubella syndrome. J. Pediat. *71:* 665 (1967).

Smetana, H. F. and Johnson, F. B.: Neonatal jaundice with giant cell transformation of the hepatic parenchyma. Am. J. Pediat. *31:* 747 (1955).

Sotgiu, G.: Post-grad. méd. J. *41:* 234 (1965); cit. With (chap. 1).

Steiner, J. W.; Carruthers, J. S., and Kalifat, S. R.: Expl. molec. Path. *1:* 162
and 427 (1962); cit. With (chap. 1).

Strauss, L. and Bernstein, L.: Neonatal hepatitis in congenital rubella: a histopathological study. Archs Path. *86:* 317 (1968).

Sulzer, W. W. and Brown, A. K.: Neonatal jaundice. Am. J. Dis. Child. *101:* 87
(1961).

Szentpétery, R.: Über die congenitale Atresie der extrahepatischen Gallengänge.
Zentbl. Chir. *89:* 553 (1964).

Visakorpi, J. K. and Sulamaa, M.: Obstructive jaundcie in ealry infancy. Annls
Paediat. Fenn. *10:* 203 (1964).

Warren, T. W.; Athanasiades, S. y Monge, I.: in Horton Vesícula biliar y con-
ductos biliares. Med. Annu. *26:* 619 (1968).

Weller, T. H. and Hanshaw, J. B.: Virological and clinical observations on cytomegalic inclusion disease. New Engl. J. Med. *266:* 1233 (1962).

Welte, W.: Diagnostische und therapeutische Probleme bei der Gallengangsatresie.
Dt. med. Wschr. *96:* 899 (1971).

Wood, R. L.: An electron microscopic study of developing bile canaliculi in rat.
Anat. Rec. *151:* 435 (1966).

Chapter 4

Establishing a Definitive, or
Absolutely Sure Diagnosis of Each Entity of the Triad

I. Definitive Diagnosis

It has already been stated (p. 56) that with the combination of cho-
langiography-liver biopsy only a *very probable diagnosis* can be reached.
How, then, in life a correct, sure, *definitive*[14] *diagnosis* ['Ultimate diagnosis' of HAYS *et al.*, 1967, chap. 1] can be established? The guidelines offered by the above-mentioned authors with some of our own suggestions
may be followed:

1. *A definitive diagnosis of extrahepatic biliary atresia* is reached in
those children who fulfill the following criteria: (a) they show jaundice of
obstructive type from the neonatal period; (b) they present an extrahepatic biliary system, transformed into solid cords, that do not allow one to
perform an intestinal anastomosis at the time of laparotomy; (c) in such
patients, a patent duct going from the liver to the intestine cannot be
demonstrated either by surgical exploration, by cholangiography, or in the
postmortem examination; (d) the survival time of these children is quite
long, averaging 19 months, and (e) the jaundice in these cases remains
without variation until death.

The diagnosis of extrahepatic biliary atresia may be accepted in cases
of operated neonatal obstructive jaundice where a subhepatic cyst was
found and an anastomosis performed, obtaining passage of bile into the
bowel, followed by a decrease in blood bilirubin levels and a subsequent
clinical recovery.

2. *A definitive diagnosis of neonatal hepatitis* is established in the
cases conforming to the following features:

---

14   Which requires following the evolution of the patient.

a) Presentation of a 'syndrome of neonatal hepatitis' manifested by a persistent jaundice which started within the first 4 weeks of life; hepatic disease of an obstructive type may be demonstrated by means of liver function analysis and urine and faeces examinations. With these data, other causes of jaundice, such as hemolysis, toxic diseases, sepsis, and local infection may be ruled out.

b) A patent but not dilated extrahepatic biliary system reaching from the liver to the duodenum must be demonstrated.

c) The presence of a certain amount of giant cell transformation in the parenchyma may be accepted in 'neonatal hepatitis'.

In this group of neonatal hepatitis are included those patients with obstructive jaundice from the newborn period in which the following circumstances occur: (1) At surgery, cord-like ducts were demonstrated, as in a case of atresia, preventing the performance of an anastomosis, but with eventual disappearance of the jaundice. (2) An anicteric course for at least three years has been observed. The presence of cirrhosis does not exclude the patients from this group.

It still has to be decided whether the cases of 'hereditary recurring cholestasis from birth', recently reported by AAGENAES et al. [1968] should be accepted as classical neonatal hepatitis or should be considered as a special entity. In these cases, the disease initiates at birth and giant cells are found in the biopsy specimens. Nevertheless, there are two distinctive features: the disease last for several years and can recur. Although the microscopic pathology in these cases offers nothing more than the features of neonatal hepatitis, the mentioned clinical facts set them apart from common neonatal hepatitis.

3. The establishment of a *definitive diagnosis of intrahepatic biliary atresia* is based on: (a) A prolonged clinical course, usually with a moderate jaundice with clinical signs of retention of bile acids and other lipids; maintained high levels of retention lead to the production of xanthomata. Certain characteristic somatic features in these patients (p. 19) have been recently reported by ALAGILLE et al. [1969, chap. 1]. (b) A very marked ductipenia with scarce or no inflammatory signs.

It has not been well clarified whether jaundice due to 'familial intrahepatic cholestasis', or Byler's disease, of which JUBERG et al. [1966, chap. 1] have recently reported some cases, and GRAY and SAUNDERS [1966, chap. 2] have described a malignant form, should be considered as a form of intrahepatic atresia or as an independent disease. JUBERG et al. [1966, chap. 1] believe that it should not be assimilated to intrahepatic atresia precisely because the ducts offer only minimal or no changes; they even point out that their cases differ from those of AHRENS *et al.* [1951, chap. 1] which probably are typical forms of intrahepatic atresia. Nevertheless, SHARP *et al.* [1967b, chap. 1] do believe that all these cases fall into intrahepatic atresia because some of them show a clear ductipenia. With regard to this debate, it may be noted that the cases with malignant features of GRAY and SAUNDERS [1966, chap. 2] show normal ducts, and these authors believe that in this case with poor prognosis two physio-pathological aspects are present: a glucurinization error and a deficiency in the elimination of conjugated elements.

II. Absolutely Sure Diagnosis

An unquestionable and *absolutely sure* diagnosis can only be made after a detailed macroscopic and microscopic study of the liver and bile ducts. This seems to be a logical assertion. However, the pathological study has not always solved the diagnostic problem. In a case from HAYS *et al.* [1967, chap. 1] in which two surgical biopsies and two cholangiographies were performed, an unquestionable diagnosis could not be reached and the postmortem study could not offer a diagnosis either. Could this case be dismissed as only a chance observation? Or should it be considered as a proof of the limitations of our present knowledge and techniques? Considering the preceding discussion, we are inclined to think that this is very likely a mixed case of atresia and hepatitis.

References

AAGENAES, O.; HAGEN, C. B. VAN DEN, and REFSUM, S.: Hereditary recurrent cholestasis from birth. Archs Dis. Childh. *43:* 646 (1968).

Chapter 5

Pathogenic Unity of the Entities of the Triad

The correlation between hepatitis and atresia has been pointed out by several authors. One of the earliest reports is the paper by SCOTT *et al.* [1954, chap. 2] about three brothers with neonatal hepatitis, one of them with concomitant atresia of the extrahepatic ducts. Two other siblings and the mother showed pathological hepatic tests.

These authors suggest that neonatal hepatitis and atresia constitute two pathological manifestations caused by the same agent, indicating the possibility that the one responsible for neonatal hepatitis could cause a malformation of the bile ducts if acting in the first 3 months of intrauterine life.

Other papers on the same subject followed [PETERMAN, 1957; STRANSKY and LARA, 1960]. In a very interesting paper, SILVERBERG *et al.* [1960, chap. 1], report two cases of extrahepatic atresia where the microscopic image was that of hepatitis with giant cells; and in a review of 260 cases of extrahepatic atresia and 38 of neonatal hepatitis, plus 80 clinical files, they found two cases of atresia where the diagnosis of hepatitis was ruled out with great difficulty and two other cases with gross pathology of atresia where it was not possible to decide whether the microscopic appearance corresponded to hepatitis or to atresia. Discussing the various possible explanations for these cases, the authors advanced the opinion that a single agent is capable of producing both diseases, although they pointed out at that time (1960) that there was no satisfactory explanation for the simultaneous occurrence of hepatitis and atresia. These authors, as most contemporary and previous authors, accept as a matter of fact that atresia is due to an embryogenic disorder, ascribed by BÖHM [1913], many years ago, to a failure in the recanalization of the ducts, an opinion accepted by no less an authority than YLPPÖ [1913, chap. 1].

In the last years, the concept of a narrow interrelation between hepatitis and atresia has gained ground, thanks to the work of SMETANA *et al.*

[1965, chap. 2], ALAGILLE [1965, chap. 2], GUBERN-SALISACHS [1968, 1971], JONES *et al.* [1968, chap. 1] etc. and very recently LANDING [1974].

But as early as 1962 PICKETT wrote: 'It is quite obvious that there exists no decisive differentiation between the cases which show a gigantic-cellular reaction and those with anatomical obstruction due to atresia.'

Nevertheless, it was PROCHIANTZ [1962, chap. 2] who expressed in a more outspoken fashion the unitarian concept of these processes, considering the paradoxical pathological and clinical correlations in a number of cases; this idea, which at the beginning found little echo, has gained many followers as of late.

To prove it, we may quote HAYS *et al.* [1967, chap. 1]: Many of the findings in the revision of a material based on 108 cases with a precise diagnosis of hepatitis or atresia (i.e. an 'ultimate' diagnosis) 'are consistent with the hypothesis that these disorders represent different phases of the same fundamental process, as well as with the hypothesis that these disorders result from a common reaction of the tissues to several different kinds of injurious factors'.

In our opinion, there are three main reasons to explain why the unitarian concept has hardly been considered, or even neglected by the vast majority of authors:

1. The great pathological-clinical difference, much more in the pathological than in the clinical aspects, between one and the other. In the first, the large bile ducts are visible, or at least patent; in the other, they are so deteriorated that in the majority of cases they have been reduced to mere traces, if they have not totally disappeared. The therapeutic possibilities offer also a great diversity; an essentially medical treatment is advocated in neonatal hepatitis, while extrahepatic atresia is susceptible of being treated only by surgical methods.

2. The pathogenic assumption of dysembryogeny as a manifestation of a dysgerminal etiology, as the cause of atresia, has been admitted year after year by the majority of authors.

This concept was upheld, even very recently, by such noted authors as STOWENS [1959, chap. 1; 1963; 1966, chap. 2] and SMETANA *et al.* [1965, chap. 2]. This judgement, defended by so many authorities, is understandably highly respected; few authors have dared to maintain that a noxa acting after the organogenetic period could be held responsible. The denomination of biliary hypoplasia [PORTER *et al.*, 1968] in cases with ducts of diminished size and/or absent, with associated malformations, emphatically suggests a dysontogenic determinism; and it seems it would not be reasonable to advocate, in these cases, another pathogenesis. This dysembryological theory was also accepted because its 'challenging' hepatitis was thought – according to a general consensus of opinion – to be an acquired infection acting in the course of the fetal period.

3. The impossibility of experimentally proving, up to recently, the etiological assumption of the acquired cause, and the suspicion that a hepatitic virus could be the responsible agent for the great majority of cases currently sustained on very solid grounds defied etiological comprobation not knowing the virus or an animal susceptible to it.

At the present moment, the possibility of its identification by means of innoculation into marmosets [HOLMES *et al.*, 1966; KÖHLER and APODACA, 1968; APODACA *et al.*, 1968] has opened the way to undertaking an etiological investigation of this problem.

I. The Triad Entities as Pathogenic Expression of a Destructive-Inflammatory Process

This section deals with fundamental data on which the unitarian pathogenical concept is based.

1. The observation of cases in families where one offered the characteristics of atresia and another those of hepatitis: The observations of SCOTT *et al.* [1954, chap. 2], GUBERN-SALISACHS [1971], ALAGILLE *et al.* [1969, chap. 1] are good examples of this situation. The later authors reported their observation of two cases of intrahepatic atresia, one of extrahepatic atresia, and another of hepatitis in four siblings.

2. The existence of cases evolving from one entity to another: The prolonged follow-up observation of some cases has uncovered many examples of partial or clear change from one entity to another.

We may point out the evolution in some cases of neonatal hepatitis towards intrahepatic atresia referred by ANDERSEN [chap. 3], GHADIMI [chap. 3], ALAGILLE [1965, chap. 2], DANKS [1965, chap. 1], and the observations of GUBERN-SALISACHS [1968, 1971] which gave ground to his conception of 'La maladie atrésiante des voies biliaires extrahépatiques'. In a wide sense, the reports by some authors who have witnessed the recovery of patency of ducts, previously seen in atretic state, could also be considered as transitional cases, or at least as an index of the regenerative capacity of the excretory system.

3. The contingency of the pathological diagnosis, which depends on the truthfulness of the microscopic appearance: We have discussed quite extensively in chapter 2.VI the problems posed by the mixed, particular or 'erroneous' cases. The demonstration of the very frequent mixed cases, with microscopic appearance corresponding to two entities of the triad in

the same patient constitutes, as we see it, a very valuable argument on which to found a unitarian pathogeny.

If *only* pure cases of inflammation or atresia would be found there would be no doubt that even accepting one single etiology capable of producing them, a different pathogenesis, should be admitted for each of them. But if we consider the existence of cases with simultaneous occurrence of inflammatory changes and atresia in the same patient, as a careful observation abundantly shows, although one of the pictures usually prevails, we believe that it will have to be admitted that both manifestations recognize the same origin or a *comon* pathogenesis: an inflammatory and destructive disease, which in some cases, due to a major intensity of the deleterious effect, or due to the fact of not being followed by a complete regeneration, leaves as sequelae a hypotrophy or complete atrophy of the excretory system, manifested by a decrease or disappearance of the lumen of the ducts, which is precisely the etimological meaning of *atresia*.

4. Last but not least: *In each of the entities,* there are more or less intense *signs* of disease of the liver gland and its excretory structures, *which reveal a histopathogenesis* that even presenting particular characters, *is fundamentally the same.* Its three most outstanding features are: a process of d-d-n, peculiar reactional dynamics, and the d-d-n process affecting also the regenerated and proliferated structures.

The concept of the pathogenic unity has prompted us to consider the reasons for the prevalence of features usually leading to a definite entity.

Not considering the possibility of an interpretation aimed towards classifying every case in a well-defined group or entity, as could be justified by reasons of synthesis or taxonomy, two possibilities should be considered: (1) Is it due to the particular disposition of the liver structures? (2) Does it really depend on the specificity of the injurious agent?

These are difficult questions to answer. We know, however, that from an epidemiologic point of view, every pathological manifestation involves a correlation between the injurious agent and the individual susceptibility to it. That is to say, the pathological effect always constitutes the expression of the result of this correlation. In chapter 6, where the etiological problem is considered, this important question is discussed.

II. Further on the Scarce Consideration which up to Recently Has Been Given to the Unipathogenic Conception of the Triad

Why have the majority of authors, both clinicians and pathologists, considered for a long time these three entities, and very especially extrahepatic atresia and neonatal hepatitis, as different from each other and without any relation among them?

We believe this latter and most important question may be easily answered by considering the way these processes have been traditionally conceived. For instance, even in very recent papers, extrahepatic atresia has been considered *pathogenically* as an *ontogenic* disorder: as a dysontogenic process manifested by a defect of the development (which takes place especially during the blastoembryonic period) and/or a trouble of the growth (which takes place specially during the fetal period), as *agenesia* and/or *aplasia*; while neonatal hepatitis was ascribed to a probably viral disease, occurring during the fetal life and which *pathogenically* would appear as an *inflammatory process*.

Only very recently opinions dissenting from these conceptions have begun to appear. Some of them [SMETANA *et al.*, 1965, chap. 2] have interpreted neonatal hepatitis as developmental disorder. Others, with increasing frequency, have also proffered doubts about the dysontogenical pathogenic theory of atresia, although the idea that extrahepatic atresia constitutes an acquired injury rather than a developmental disorder was already put forward by ROLLESTON and HAYNE [1901] and by FRENSDORF [1912], who pointed out that: 'The first hing would be an inflammation in some part of the liver, inflammation of an unknown but not luetic cause, which would lead to a pericholangiolithic proliferation. This tissue would compress itself inside the still tender ducts and would strangle them.'

The fact that biliary atresia constitutes a dynamic disease rather than a static, congenitally fixed process, is already mentioned in the works of KANOF *et al.* [1953, chap. 3], GROSS [1953, chap. 1], REDO [1954, chap. 3], and CARLSON [1960, chap. 3]. But these authors are so conditioned by the idea of a dysontogenic disorder that they interpret the fact that a case of atresia not amenable to surgical repair in a first intervention, should later become treatable, in the sense that the development of the ducts continues after birth.

It is especially after BRENT [1962, chap. 1] that the possibility that atresia could be the result of the destruction of some already formed bile ducts rather than a malformation is stressed[15].

BLANC, in an enquiry carried out by the mentioned author, sustains

---

15 Already conceived by AHRENS *et al.* [1951, chap. 1] although they clearly lean towards a dysontogenical interpretation.

with good arguments the possibility of the late inflammatory obliteration of the ducts.

To back his concept he argues: (1) Few facts are offered by traditional embryology to support the hypothesis of a lack of segmentation in the formation of ducts. (2) He never saw a well-documented case of atresia either in autopsies of fetuses who died before birth or in premature babies. (3) In two cases he has demonstrated an inflammatory process with progressive obliteration of the extrahepatic ducts in surgical specimens of the hilum taken from an area where they were not microscopically visible. (4) In the autopsy specimens of the hilar area, fibrous sequelae of bile ducts, in form of cords, are found. (5) The disappearance of the lumen of the ducts can be the consequence of an inflammation.

To these arguments of BLANC BRENT adds the following: (1) There has not been up to now any constant observation of clay-like feces in patients who suffer from biliary atresia. (2) Extrahepatic biliary atresia is as rare as intestinal atresia in experimental teratological studies. We have not seen such lesions in experimental animals submitted to teratogenical agents during the organogenetical period. BRENT goes on to say:

SCOTT et al. [1954, chap. 2] postulated that a viral disease can induce biliary atresia in utero, acting in a fashion similar to that of rubella, i.e. dysontogenically. Incidentally, this was the pathogenic mechanism considered at that time, and presently as responsible for cataracts, coclear disorders, etc. But, it could also occur, BRENT points out, as we have already indicated, that the injury to the biliary tree occurs as a complication of neonatal hepatitis. The available evidence (1962) is not sufficient to affirm or deny an etiological relation between hepatitis and atresia.

This point has not been completely resolved for all the cases at present (1974). Nevertheless, such a relationship seems to be demonstrated for the case in which the causal agent is the rubella virus, and a great number of arguments already exists for admitting that a similar thing occurs with the hepatitis virus.

KAYE et al. [1957] and HOLDER [1964] pointed out the apparent development of postnatal atresia. In the last years, a good number of authors [ISHIDA et al., 1965; HAI-CHIN-CHEN, 1965; TER-GRIGOROWA, 1965; DANKS and CAMPBELL, 1966, chap. 2; GUBERN-SALISACHS, 1968; HAYS et al., 1967, chap. 1] defended the concept of an acquired etiology, expressed pathogenically as an inflammatory-destructive process, as opposed to the classical one of the germinal plasma etiology and dysontogenical pathogenesis. As NEGRO and LARGUERO [1965, chap. 3] pertinently indicate, an added inflammatory obstruction later in the fetal period can constitute the first logical explanation for the presence of bile-stained fecal material in the patients with atresia during their first days of life.

Nevertheless, the pathogenic concept of the developmental disorder has prevailed for such a long time that it deserves further discussion. By disproving such a concept, the hypothesis of an inflammatory destructive pathogenesis will logically be strengthened; this will also constitute another valid point in favor of the unitarian pathogenic conception of the triad.

III. Discussion of the Dysembryological Conception of the Entities of the Triad

Some type of ontogenical disturbance has been considered responsible for both intrahepatic and extrahepatic atresia, and particularly so for the latter, where larger ducts are involved. Intrahepatic atresia, on the other hand, was soon considered as an acquired disorder by a good number of authors.

Too much emphasis has been laid by the clinicians when dealing with this problem on an embryological approach, not always offered in a clearly outlined fashion. Embryological hypotheses or theories rather than unquestionable facts have been persistently used in the pathogenic interpretation of the pathology in the entities we are discussing.

A. Extrahepatic Atresia

During the long time in which the malformations were considered, with few exceptions, as alterations of the germinal plasma, since THOMSON [1891–92], BÖHM [1913], and YLPPÖ [1913, chap. 1], atresia was considered as a disorder of dysgenic etiology, pathogenically manifested by a dysontogeny.

The dysontogenical conception has been variously interpreted as a developmental arrest [STOWENS, 1963; SMETANA et al., 1965, chap. 2], as a major embryological defect, considering the great extension of the lesions [MOORE, 1953, chap. 1], or in the oldest and most commonly held concept, as a recanalization defect of the ducts. Let us consider with a certain detail the theoretical explanations offered to back this last pathogenic interpretation, which for a long time has been little less than an article of faith.

It has been maintained that in a period of the embryological organogenesis, the bile ducts, initially developed as hollow structures, undergo a process of *epithelial hyperplasia* to become compact cords, or adopt a 'solid state'; later on, each of these cords will be recanalized. When the recanalization process is disturbed, due to a failure in the reabsorption of the proliferated elements or to an incomplete vacuolization of the structures, etc. [BÖHM, 1913; YLPPÖ, 1913, chap. 1; RIETZ, 1917; LADD and GROSS, 1941, chap. 2; SHERLOCK[16], 1971, chap. 2], the organogenesis of the ducts is altered, with ductal atresia as the end result.

According to RIETZ [1917], the resulting type of atresia would be determined by the moment when the disturbance of the development takes place. When it occurs in a 9-mm embryo, a total atresia is the result; if it affects an 11-mm embryo, atresia will only affect the hepatic duct; atresia of the cystic duct and gallbladder is the result of a developmental alteration in 11- to 14-mm embryos, whereas atresia limited to the gallbladder would correspond to a failure in the development occurring in a 30-mm embryo.

CAMERON and BUNTON [1960, chap. 1] described the outstanding fact that in atresia the meconium appears colored. In the 6-week embryo, the liver starts its hematopoietic activity, which reaches its maximum towards the fifth month. At 12 weeks, the liver secretes bile. As in other tubular structures of the embryo, the *hyperplasia* of the epithelium obstructs the lumen of the ducts around the fourth month, but their recanalization is completed by the fifth month. In atresia, the first meconium is of normal color because it was secreted by the fourth month and it was of a normal green color.

Thus, extrahepatic atresia has been considered for many years and by noted authors basically as an embryological disorder. To the already mentioned authors, we may quote, as sustaining this point of view, OBERNIEDERMAYER [1959], REHBEIN and NEWMANN [1957], VEGHELY [1964][17], and others. On this subject, RAPAPORT [1950, 1959] deserves special mention; he very specifically indicates that this is a developmental arrest, ruling out any inflammatory cuase as no symptoms of fetal peritonitis or syphilis have ever been demonstrated. Some authors, for example GOHRBRANDT et al. [1928] and GROB [1957], take a more eclectic view, admitting that the disorder may also be due on occasion to an inflammatory process which would occur in the later fetal period.

The dysontogenic theory of recanalization failure to explain the atresia of the extrahepatic ducts is a faithful replica of the one offered by TANDLER [1902] and continued by JOHNSON [1910] and by KREUTER [KLEINSCHMIDT, 1931] to explain the atresia of the gut.

According to these authors, the epithelial excrescences which occur in the lumen of the intestine between the 30th and 60th day of life are causes of atresia due to an evolutionary defect. Even in 1964, DUHAMEL and HAEGEL admit that an organogenesis disturbance of the alimentary canal, in accordance with TANDLER's

16 In the new edition of her book, SHERLOCK still maintains the following point of view: 'The majority of congenital anomalies can be related to alterations in the original budding from the foregut or to failure of vacuolization of the solid gallbladder and bile diverticulum.'
17 Adopting the name of aplasia.

[1902] concept, seems plausible enough to explain the majority of constitutional anomalies of the bowel. They add, though, that this is no presumption about the primary cause of this embryogenic disturbance.

Nevertheless, for many years, serious doubts have been voiced against this dysembryogenic theory to explain the atresia of the gut based on an observation constituting an argument of great importance: the presence, in these cases of atresia, of normal meconium [SCHRIEDE, cit. KLEINSCHMIDT, 1931]. Evidently, it seems impossible that the meconium can show its normal greeny-black color if the intestinal lumen was blocked before the bile excretion by the liver takes place (sect. IIIA.1, this chapter).

Serious objections of this theory have also been raised by other authors. ROUVIÈRE points out that in the extensive series of human embryos he had studied, he never came across a case of pathological epithelial obstruction; DUHAMEL [1956] likewise points out that TANDLER's [1902] theory lies on equivocal bases, and CARPENTER [1962] states that the theory of the lack of epithelial recanalization is missing in convincing facts and that the infrequent association of intestinal atresia with other congenial malformations is further evidence against the hypothesis of an embryological malformation.

The recent embryologic studies in humans by MOUTSOURIS [1967] are an excellent contribution to disprove the dysembriologic concept of intestinal atresia.

According to this author, the primitive intestine is already well-defined and with a normal lumen by the fifth week. Later on, between the sixth and seventh weeks, the lumen of the duodenum becomes partially filled by epithelial elements which do not totally occlude it, as vacuoles are found among them; he has been unable to find any epithelial hyperplasia of this type outside the duodenum.

These studies confirm our point of view that a physiological epithelial hyperplasia within tubular structures can be perhaps totally obstructive only when the mucosa lining is arranged in multiple folds, e.g. in the duodenum[18] or in narrower tubular structures, e.g. the large bile ducts, where the mucosa shows cripts.

We believe it is reasonable to admit that, both in the duodenum and

18   The duodenal mucosa shows transversal folds (plicae circulares) or connivent valves, which 'are lacking in its initial portion'. They appear in the second portion and acquire a greater development in the following two portions and in the proximal jejunal loops. Further down, these plicae become gradually smaller and scattered further apart to entirely disappear in the final segment of the small bowel, 60–80 cm above the ileocecal valve [TESTUT and LATARJET, 1944].

in the large bile ducts, and at a given moment of its development, the mucosa layer grows actively under the influence of a connective inductor within the lumen and partially or perhaps totally occludes it. The growth of the middle layer of the structure, corresponding mainly to muscular tissue, enlarges the diameter of the organ and reestablishes completely its patency.

Referring to this process as a recanalization of the ducts it seems to make the development of a patent lumen dependent on such an epithelial growth, when what really occurs is that the lumen is restored when the organ attains larger dimensions due mainly to the growth of its middle, mesenchymal layer. If the epithelium invades the lumen at a certain moment of the embryonic development, it will be due to a slower growth of the middle layer, as it usually occurs.

We believe that it is not possible to assert or deny that the lesions which constitute the substratum of atresia should originate by this epithelial hyperplasia, because the end result is offered to our observation in extrauterine life a long time after such an embryological event. What we can assert, nevertheless, is that atresia simply due to epithelial growth (which would not be atresia then, but simply obstruction) would never occur. No one has ever described a case where this epithelial growth had been observed – quite the contrary. The structure of the ducts is always found to be so altered that it is sometimes difficult to find eventraces of them, particularly of the epithelial elements.

Added to the just mentioned arguments against the dysembryogenic hypothesis supported by so many authors, there is an observation of very significant value: the *presence of normal colored meconium in the majority of cases of atresia*. The material which stains the meconium to its characteristic deep green hue comes from the liver, and has been elaborated by the gland after the embryonic period has finished.

However, KÜNZER et al. [1965] have recently reported some cases of biliary and duodenal atresia with normal meconium and cases of intestinal atresia with abnormally colored, whitish stools. The cases reported were of total biliary or duodenal atresia; they can be considered as 'natural models of study' (or as an experiment devised by nature, one could say), where the biliary pigments *cannot* reach the distal part of the intestinal tract by the usual route of the bile ducts and the upper intestinal loops. The presence of normal meconium in such cases is interpreted by KÜNZER et al. [1965] as proof of the existence of *bilirubin that can pass directly from the blood to the intestine.*

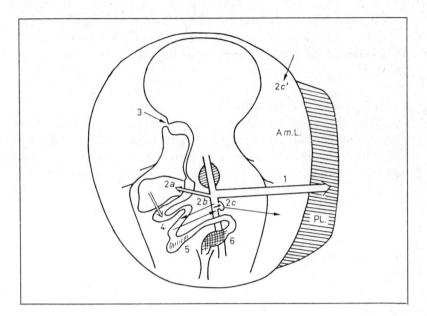

Fig. 11. Bilirubin in the fetus. (1) Placental route – through it, 24/25 of the indirect bilirubin elaborated by the fetus is excreted; (2a) hepatobiliary route; (2b) intestinal route; (2c) renal route; (2c') amniotic route, with the previous one it will carry bilirubin to the amniotic fluid, from which it will pass to the (3) oral route; (4) intestinal resorption route; (5) not reabsorbed bilirubin which will keep on accumulating in the meconium; (6) meconium. 2a, 2b, 2c, 3, and 4 constitute the 'blood-digestive tract-blood' circle. Bilirubin in the fetus.

Therefore, following these authors, as the coloring of the meconium in atresia might be due to the bilirubin excreted by this route, we must reconsider the dysembryological pathogeny, as the demonstration of its unlikelihood requires further discussion.

There is a good number of reasons that have convinced us of the fact that *a normal or abnormal meconium cannot recognize any other inter-pretation than the different timing in the production of the originating le-sion,* i.e. the moment in intrauterine life when this narrowing or atresia-inducing process takes place (see conclusions deduced from the physiology of the pigmentation of the meconium, p. 125) very probably without any relation to the alleged intestinal route of bilirubin elimination.

As our reasoning is based precisely in the 'production' of the pigmentation of the meconium, this significant bilogical fact deserves a detailed consideration.

A) Physiology of the Meconium Pigmentation

The pigmentation of the meconium is involved in the dynamics of the metabolism of the fetal bilirubin and is depicted in a schematic drawing (fig. 11).

1. Dynamics of Fetal Bilirubin

No direct measurements or accurate values of the elements theoretically responsible for the staining of the meconium are available at present, and it will surely be a long time before these determinations are carried out due less to technical difficulties than to the barriers imposed by ethics to the experimentation on human subjects. Nevertheless, indirect, approximate data on the elements of this circle are available; in the present state of our knowledge they enable us to understand and evaluate with reasonable precision the dynamics of the fetal bilirubin. These concepts, if not absolutely proven, must certainly be quite close to the real facts concerning the process of pigmentation of the meconium.

a) If it is accepted that metabolism in fetal life is quantitatively and qualitatively similar to that of extrauterine life, it would follow that the total amount of bilirubin mostly produced in the catabolic breakdown of hemoglobin by the fetus until the end of its intrauterine life should amount to 1,000 mg [BETKE, 1959].

b) From this amount, YLPPÖ [1913] states that in the meconium of the newborn at term there are 33 mg, while in seventh-month, premature babies, only 3.9 mg are found. These figures are the sum of bilirubin and biliverdin determined simultaneously and independently.

c) The bile pigment in the meconium is made of bilirubin, especially in its conjugated form, and also biliverdin[19]. The importance of this oxidated bilirubin should not be overlooked, because as YLPPÖ [1913] indicated, a great part (often half and sometimes more) of the meconial pigment is biliverdin.

This assertion of the Finnish author has later on been confirmed by other authors: LARSEN and WITH [1943] studied the composition of the meconial pigments in 23 newborns using the dyazoic method, which does not detect biliverdin. They found a small amount of bilirubin in most cases and in 10 they did not see any traces of it. Likewise, HERINGOVÁ et al. [1964] found 7 out of 21 cases with a negative diazoic reaction, the other 14 only presenting conjugated bilirubin. The fact that in the composition of the pigments of the meconium biliverdin plays a very im-

19 Derived from bilirubin and probably from the direct one secreted by the liver, taking into account that it occurs like this in postuterine life.

portant role is also pointed out in the studies of GARAY et al. [1964] who, in 50 samples of meconium, found that this pigment figures in the proportion of 64% (paper cromatography).

d) The authors show remarkable differences in their estimates of pigment found in the meconium.

These are probably related to individual variations in biological parameters and to the various methods of study. Marked differences also exist, however, even when using identical methods of determination.

FASHENA [1948], obtained by the oxidative method of EVELYN and MALLOY, which gives the sum of bilirubin and biliverdin.

Cases	Serum bilirubin mg%	Pigment in 100 g meconium[1], mg	Average pigment mg
6	5	25–102	58.5
6	5–10	16–62	33.7
8	> 10	12–37	26

1 The amount of meconium of a newborn at term normally fluctuates between 70 and 90 g.

VEST [1959] gives the following figures:

Cases	Serum bilirubin levels, mg%	Meconium	
		bilirubin + biliverdin content (average) mg	urobilin content (average) mg
11	0–5	29.40	1.24
16	5–10	17.43	0.85
14	10–15	13.79	0.70
4	15–25	7.66	0.33

Note that, apart from the curious fact that the amount of meconial pigment is in an inverse proportion to the serum blood bilirubin levels [VEST, 1959], the figures of FASHENA [1948] are higher than those of YLPPÖ [1913], whereas those of VEST [1959] are lower. As the figures given by YLPPÖ [1913] for the amount of bile pigment in the meconium of a newborn at term are intermediate between the previous ones, this figure and the one given by the same author for premature babies (p. 114) will be used in the speculative considerations that follow. The values given by YLPPÖ [1913] will not be taken as exact figures, but will be rounded as follows: 30–35 mg as the sum of bilirubin and biliverdin present in the meconium of a newborn at term, and 4 mg as the figure of the same pigments in the premature of about 7 months.

e) The indicated estimated amounts of bile pigments present in the meconium suggest that only 1/25 of the fetal bilirubin is found in the meconium. The other 24/25 parts will have been eliminated, destroyed or both. It is generally accepted that the greater part of fetal bilirubin that has not passed into the feces is eliminated by the placenta. Various facts guarantee this conception.

1. FINDLEY et al. [1947], in 23 newborn babies, found that the bilirubin levels in the blood in the umbilical artery was 14% higher by average than the one in the vein, which indicates that a certain amount of bilirubin has passed from the placenta to the maternal ciculation.

2. Recent experimental studies with radioisotope-labeled bilirubin have modified the classical idea expressed especially by YLPPÖ [1913] that fetal bilirubin does not pass into the placental barrier. In effect, SHENKER et al. [1964] have demonstrated in guinea pigs that ^{14}C-bilirubin injected in the fetal circulation is promptly carried to the mother's bloodstream. This form of excretion occurs especially with *unconjugated* bilirubin and only in a small proportion with the conjugated fraction. As albumin does not pass into the placenta, it must be accepted that during the transfer process the bilirubin binding to albumin must be broken. Similar observations have been carried out in pregnant monkeys [LESTER et al., 1963], suggesting that the excretion of bilirubin by the placenta takes also place in the human species. It is precisely to this placental excretion of bilirubin that the absence of a significant increase of the bilirubin levels in the umbilical cord blood of newborns with a hemolytic disease and its rapid increase during the first 24 h after birth must be attributed [OSKI and NAIMAN, 1966].

f) The bilirubin (and with it the biliverdin) of the meconium can theoretically recognize the following origins:

1. *Oral ingestion* of amniotic fluid, where bilirubin comes from two sources: one corresponding to the secretion of the ovum membranes and another contributed by the urinary excretion of the fetus.

2. *Hepatic secretion.* From the third month onwards, bile is found in the gallbladder [ZWEIFEL, 1875]. AREY [1946] also says that the liver secretes from the fourth month on and SMITH [1970] equally accepts as an established fact that bile is produced in the twelfth week (8.8-cm embryo) and meconium in the 16th week (14-cm fetus).

3. A possible *intestinal excretion* (see p. 112). This would take place perhaps not as a transudate, but as a true excretion.

Part of the bilirubin reaching the gut undergoes an intestinal resorption, but the remaining proceeds down the intestinal tract, accumulating in the distal segments where it joints with other excretions to form the meconium and stain it.

In summary, the pigmentation of the meconium depends intrinsically on the dynamics of the 'blood-digestive tract-blood' circle of bilirubin, although the data we have about it are too scarce to provide a completely defined picture.

Against the time-honored concept that the pigment elaborated by the liver is secreted through the bloodstream [LEREBOULLET] and that the presence of normally colored meconium beyond an intestinal obstacle may be readily explained by the pigment transport through the blood [DUHAMEL, 1956], it may be argued that *there are many reasons to admit the predominant, if not exclusive role of the hepatic excretion*, as we shall see immediately.

2. Hepatic Secretion as a Source of the Bile Pigment of the Meconium
a) Facts Militating against the Importance of Other Sources of Bile Pigment for the Meconium

Oral ingestion. One *capital* argument, as current knowledge seems to prove, against the meconium being stained by the bilirubin present in the amniotic liquid lies in the fact that *there are a few cases of atresia and neonatal hepatitis with colorless meconium* (as already mentioned on p. 17). In these cases, no gross pathology suggesting a functional alteration of the digestive tract has been found; should the coloring of the meconium depend on the pigment ingested by the fetus, no reasonable explanation could be offered for these cases with colorless meconium. Let us consider this problem with some detail:

Starting at the fourth month of intrauterine life, the fetus swallows more and more amniotic fluid. According to ROSA [1951], towards the end of pregnancy the amount can be rated at about 500 ml per day, i.e. during the 9 months the fetal body ingests some 12 liters of this fluid. According to MACKAY and WATSON [1962], the amniotic fluid usually contains throughout the 33 weeks of pregnancy between 0.00 and 0.11 mg% of bilirubin (azoic method)[20]. A simple calculation will show that by the ninth month, accepting a maximal concentration, the total fetus intake can reach up to 13 mg of bilirubin. Adding to this the intake of the previous month and that accumulated throughout the whole course of pregnancy up to the end of the seventh or beginning of the eighth month [some 4 mg of bilirubin and biliverdin, according to YLPPÖ, 1913] the total fetal intake may amount up to approximately 25 mg of bilirubin. This quantity could certainly produce a good coloring of the meconium, knowing that between 30 and 35 mg of bilirubin may give the meconium its normal hue.

This would only be the case if maximal concentrations of bilirubin in the amniotic fluid were present. Nevertheless, in a good number of cases, the bilirubin lev-

20   Between 0.00 and 0.07 mg% according to data by FLEMING and WOOLF [1965], using the spectrophotometric method.

els in amniotic fluid vary from 0.0 and 0.05 mg; these amounts would signify a scant contribution of bilirubin to the meconium, causing little or no staining. Moreover, the peak of bilirubin levels in the amniotic fluid is reached between the 16th and 30th weeks; afterwards, it decreases to nil by the 36th week [MANDELBAUM *et al.*, 1967; CHERRY, 1967, and others, and recently confirmed by ANDREWS, 1970]. Thus, by the time the meconium attains a deeper pigmentation the bilirubin concentration in the amniotic fluid drops to its lowest level.

Conclusions: In some *normal cases*, the pigmentation of the meconium may be due to the ingested bilirubin, but in a good number of other instances this mechanism is obviously incapable of accounting for the staining of the meconial matter. Practically in all cases, the meconium exhibits its characteristic dark green color. This certainly makes the hypothesis of ingested bilirubin as the primary source of pigment for the meconium clearly untenable.

Similarly, *in cases of atresia or hepatitis*, the coloring of the meconium by ingested bilirubin seems to be quite unlikely. Actually, to accept such a mechanism would imply that: in the cases with normally stained meconium, which are the majority, the ingested bilirubin was causing the coloring, whereas in the cases with colorless meconium, a less common situation but certainly not a group of cases to be dismissed, the same mechanism failed to work. This would require one to accept the ingested bilirubin staining the meconium in some cases and not doing it in some others. Is it possible that some fetuses act with one physiology and others with a completely different one? It seems that the possibilities of this occurring are very remote.

According to the preceding reasoning, if the ingested indirect bilirubin does not contribute in a predominant fashion to the pigmentation of the meconium in all likelihood, *it must be absorbed* through the intestinal wall, as is known to occur in extrauterine life, both in humans and rats, as LESTER and SCHMID [1963] have demonstrated by means of studies with ^{14}C-labeled bilirubin. But only a very small proportion of conjugated bilirubin is absorbed; in its greater part it is hydrolyzed and absorbed in a free way. Then, the same happens to bilirubin as happens to other components of the amniotic fluid which are ingested: salts, urea, etc. will later follow the route of the true emunctory – the placenta.

It does not seem likely that bilirubin is destroyed, as destruction processes even in extrauterine life, when the organic catabolism is most marked, are of very little intensity. Perhaps it is partly transformed either by oxidation to biliverdin, although this eventuality is characteristic of direct bilirubin, or by reduction to urobilinogen or urobilin. For this to take place, a process different from those seen in postuterine

life, when the bilirubin reduction is carried out thanks to the activity of the intestinal flora, would be required. The newborn shows bilirubin breakdown products only
when bacterial pollution of the intestinal tract has set in. On the other hand, it must
be pointed out that the amount of reduced bilirubin in the meconium with relation
to the amount supposedly ingested is very small. According to KÜNZER [1962,
chap. 1], up to a maximum of 5 mg, and according to GARAY et al. [1964], in 50 meconium samples, an average of 3.4 μg/g, i.e. approximately 0.3 mg.

A fact apparently proving this intestinal bilirubin absorption is that the later the
elimination of the meconium takes place, the higher is the hyperbilirubinemia of the
newborn. ROSTA et al. [1968], in 125 mature newborn babies with blood bilirubin
levels above 15 mg%, in the course of the first fortnight, found that the elimination
of meconium occurred at an average 11.7 h after birth, while in a control group of
950 babies the meconium expulsion took place after 9.8 h; the difference between
the two groups is significant ($p < 1\%$). Some authors accept the inverted relationship
between the bilirubin contents of the meconium and the serum bilirubin level [see
previous data of FASHENA, 1948, and VEST, 1959] as an indication of this absorption, although a hypothetic decrease in intestinal (see below) or hepatic excretion
(p. 121) must be also considered.

Summary: *The physiological circumstance and pathological features
in hepatitis and atresia* with normally stained or colorless meconium, *appear to support the physiological fact* that an intestinal absorption of indirect bilirubin takes place in the fetus. Otherwise destruction of bilirubin
or its transformation into colorless products would have to be advocated,
a possibility ruled out by our discussion on the physiology of meconium
pigmentation.

Intestinal excretion. While the existence of an absorption process
seems quite obvious, the bilirubin secretion by the intestinal wall in physiological conditions does not appear to be so clear.

a) It seems contradictory to admit, as many authors have been doing up to
now, that a product whose elimination by the liver-biliary tract system in the course
of fetal life is progressively increased and which later in extrauterine life is practically eliminated only by the liver, can proceed from the intestinal secretion. If this
bilirubin secretion exists it must be in a minimal amount. If the hepatic secretion
present from the third month of pregnancy through the end of the seventh month
would be excluded, the intestinal secretion would contribute at most with 4 mg of
bile pigment to the meconium.

b) It is also difficult to accept that the intestine should have the role of beak-
ing down and reabsorbing bilirubin, a process that would be tantamount to recuper-
ate a bilirubin which it has previously excreted. It seems quite logical that if it is the
intestine's role to reabsorb bilirubin, it will do so because it has reached the intestine by a different route, having discarded the oral one due to the reasons recently
discussed.

c) To the conceptions admitting the staining of the meconium by the intestinal bilirubin, it must be argued, as pointed out by GUBERN-SALISACHS [1968], that in some cases of atresia the meconium is normally colored and in some others it is colorless.

d) Recent studies by KÜNZER et al. [1965], following the ideas of SCHMID and HAMMAKER [1962], seem to support this bilirubin elimination by the upper intestinal tract during fetal life (although these authors acknowledge that more cases need to be studied to definitely assert this point), offering the following observations: (1) In cases of biliary and upper intestinal or duodenal atresia, a normally stained meconium is found, whereas a colorless meconium appears in cases with lower intestinal atresia. (2) That in some deeply jaundiced newborns or small infants (either by physiological jaundice or by a hemolytic disease of the newborn), unconjugated bilirubin can be obtained in a good proportion of cases from the duodenal juice.

In spite of these arguments, KÜNZER et al. [1965] are not categoric, stating that a very important element required for accepting their theory is the lack of a deconjugation process. They point out that: (1) It cannot be denied that in the normal newborn this indirect bilirubin can originate from the liver, to be deconjugated later on within the intestinal lumen as SHIRKEY [1964] thinks. (2) They only admit as meconial pigmentation by intestinal bilirubin that observed in cases of atresia of truly embryonic origin which, according to KÜNZER et al. [1965], are those accompanied by other malformations, these being the least common observations among atresia cases, as has already been indicated (pp. 20 and 21). In our opinion, this is probably not true either, because as we will see later (pp. 126 and 141), *the presence of accompanying malformations in a case of biliary atresia does not necessarily mean that this atresia is also of an embryonic nature.*

The existence of a physiological process of deconjugation of bilirubin within the fetal intestine seems plausible, not only because this bilirubin is largely or exclusively of the deconjugated type, but also because there is an increased amount of β-glucuronidase in the newborn feces and in the meconium itself [BRODERSEN and HERMANN, 1962], noting these amounts to be significantly higher than in later ages as they decrease rapidly in successive days when the hepatic conjugation system becomes more active; COROMINAS-VILARDELL [unpublished] has corroborated these observations. POLAND and ODELL [1971] have recently considered this subject as follows: 'The absence of an intestinal bacterial flora for the reduction of bilirubin to urobilinogen and the presence of β-glucoronidase in the intestine during fetal and neonatal life presents a unique circumstance whereby bilirubin diglucuronide secreted into the intestinal tract could be hydrolyzed and the resulting bilirubin absorbed.'

There seems to be nothing against accepting that the β-glucoronidase, apart, perhaps, of other missions, would have the role of deconjugating bilirubin during the fetal period – a job which it would have to carry out in response to a physiological need. Thus, an excessive amount of conjugated bile pigment will *not* accumulate in the intestine, because this pigment and other excretions that accompany it will only be evacuated, in normal fetal conditions, in frank extrauterine life. The conjugation process, according to LESTER and SCHMID [1963], acts as a *barrier* to prevent the formation of an 'enterohepatic circle in the bilirubin of humans'.

The deconjugation of small quantities of bilirubin that have entered the intestine by the bile excretion will allow absorption of the *unconjugated* bilirubin by the distal intestinal tract to enter the circulation and follow the route towards the natural emunctory: the placenta.

e) Even assigning an intestinal origin to all the meconial pigment of a seventh-month fetus, amounting to some 4 mg (an assumption not easily justified as it has already been shown in p. 119) and admitting that for the last 2 months of pregnancy pigment will be added at a constant rate, proportional to the breakdown processes of blood elements (which in turn are dependent on weight), a simple calculation will show that the amount of bilirubin which ought to be contained in the meconium should be approximately 11 mg. But the amount normally found is much greater, about 3 times as much. Evidently, by intestinal excretion alone, a lightly teinted, abnormal-looking meconium would result. To account for the dark green coloring of the normal meconium, the presence of bilirubin of another origin will have to be admitted.

Conclusion: The possibility of a physiological excretion of bilirubin by the intestine during fetal life has only to be considered, in any case, as an accessory process of small relevance in relation to another source of secretion: the hepatobiliary one.

b) Data for the Hepatobiliary Origin of the Secretion

1. The liver offers signs of choleretic function, by the third month, as has been indicated. And this is authenticated by some observations of calcified biliary and neonatal necrosing (congenital) peritonitis in which the ovary has been found attached to the perivesicular pathological mass [MEYNADIER et al., 1970]. During the major part of the early fetal life, the biliary secretion proceeds at a slow rate significantly increasing in the late fetal period. At birth, obviously this mechanism is quite insufficient to eliminate all the hematic pigments produced by the breakdown of blood elements, a task up to then mainly performed by the placenta. This process of elimination depends basically on the conjugation of the pigments with glucuronic acid, and at birth and during the early neonatal period there is a *deficit* of the enzyme catalyzing this conjugation.

Recently, however, it has been shown that glucuronization in the newborn does not seem to be as minimal as it was thought to be. LAURITZEN and LEHMANN [1967] have pointed out that the steroid hormones such as estryol, pregnanediol, etc., but not progesterone, would have a competitive effect with bilirubin glucurinization by the liver in the newborn. In effect, the administration of such steroids to the newborn increases its blood bilirubin levels, and the same happens in small infants when these steroids are administered to the nursing mother. Therefore, one of the casues of neonatal jaundice and hyperbilirubinemia would be the large amount of steroid hormones excreted in the first days of life that have to be *previously conjugated*. A logical question arises: does the glucoryltransferase system have a greater affinity for steroid hormones than for bilirubin?

2. That the liver is functioning during fetal life and especially towards the end, although certainly less than at birth, is demonstrated by the fact that *glucoryltransferase is already found in the liver at this period*[21]. Undoubtedly, this enzyme is found in small amounts; DUTTON [1959] has found it in a negligible amount in two human fetuses of 3 and 4 months, *but it is found anyway*. Understandably, the amount to be found does not need to be even moderately important, due to the fact that at the end of the seventh month the meconium pigment only amounts to 4 mg. The amount of transferase will have to be only somewhat higher for the reason that in the course of another 2 months that figure will only increase to 30–35 mg. In 60 days, the amount of bilirubin to be elaborated equals that produced in the first 5 days after birth, when the liver is relatively insufficient [YLPPÖ, 1913]. Finally, we think it is logical to admit that the levels of fetal hepatic transpherase during the eighth and ninth months need only be exiguous to produce the small average daily amount of 0.5 mg of bilirubin, somewhat less during the eighth and more during the ninth month, especially so in the last days before the termination of pregnancy.

The idea that a bilirubin conjugating system exists with more or less intensity during fetal life, is favored by the demonstrated existence in serum of an inhibiting element of such a system. This has been found by Ko *et al.* [1967] in the chicken. Certainly, the fact of having found this inhibiting element in animals does not permit one to extrapolate its existence in the human species. WITH [1968, chap. 1] has pointed out with regard to the metabolism of bilirubin that the differences between animal species are remarkable and, as DUTTON [1959] indicates, important differences seem to exist between the glucoryltransferase of diverse animals species and that of man. These differences, which concern both the qualitative and quantitative

---

21 Assuming that the liver *only* eliminates conjugated bilirubin, of which we are not yet sure. Some authors, among them COSSEL [1965, chap. 1], believe that in extrauterine life, at least part of the indirect bilirubin of bile would proceed from hepatic secretion. The studies of HERINGOVÁ *et al.* [1964] also favor the idea that the fetal liver eliminates indirect bilirubin, because up to the 14th day after birth, when the liver function becomes obvious (cholic feces), in the majority of cases the feces contain both bilirubins, and only in a few cases just conjugated or unconjugated bilirubin. Logically, two possibilities are deduced from this; either the liver eliminates indirect bilirubin or there is a deconjugating system.

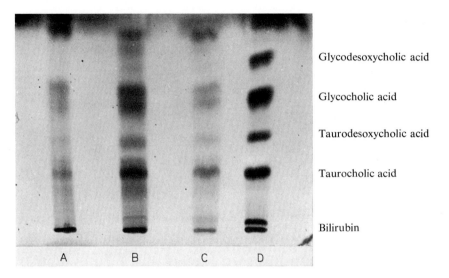

Fig. 12. Investigation of bile acids in the meconium of three newborns at term. *A* Meconium 1; *B* meconium 2; *C* meconium 3; *D* adult bile.

aspects, do not invalidate, however, the possible existence of such an inhibitor in the human species.

c) Liver Function during Fetal Life

That the liver is functioning after the seventh month in a remarkable way is proved by the demonstration in the meconium of a great amount of bile acids, easily revealed by fine-layer chromatography (fig. 12).

That the liver already is functioning, even before this time in an indisputable fashion, is also proved by the demonstration, using the same technique, that together with bilirubin, there is an appreciable amount of bile acids both in the meconium and in the contents of the gallbladder (fig. 13, 14).

We have another sign that reveals that the liver should function in a patent fashion, especially during the last 2 months, as has been already indicated (p. 123): the high figure of β-glucoronidase present in the meconium and stools of the first days of life, which later decreases rapidly in the course of a short period of time.

As is well known, the function of this enzyme is to deglucoronize. It seems that the unique substance present in the meconium that can undergo such an action is conjugated bilirubin, i.e. the bilirubin that is only se-

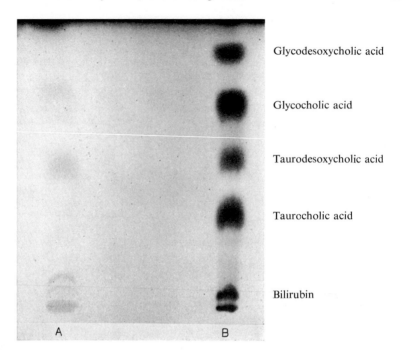

Fig. 13. Investigation of bile acids in a fetus of 6 months, weight 1,020 g. *A* Meconium; *B* adult bile. Traces of bilirubin, taurodesoxycholic acid and glycocholic acid are evident.

creted by the liver[22]. Its deconjugation and the absorption of indirect bilirubin constitute, it seems, different stages of a process designed to avoid the accumulation of bilirubin (which has laxative properties) in the meconium, a substance that is *never* evacuated, barring pathological circumstances during the hole course of fetal life; this is in contrast with the urinary excretion, which from the third month takes place into the amniotic cavity.

Should we admit that in cases with biliary atresia or hepatitis presenting an abnormal meconium the intestinal secretion of bilirubin does not take place? Why can we accept that the intestine secretes bilirubin in some fetuses and in some others it does not? It seems illogical indeed to accept such a hypothesis.

22   As has been previously mentioned (p. 120), bilirubin conjugation specifically implies that bile as an excretion is not absorbed or, at the most, only in a small proportion.

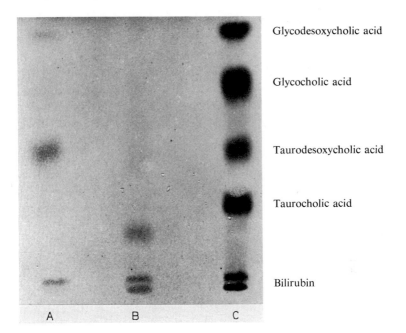

Glycodesoxycholic acid

Glycocholic acid

Taurodesoxycholic acid

Taurocholic acid

Bilirubin

A   B   C

Fig. 14. Investigation of bile acids in a fetus of 6 months, weight 1,020 g. *A* Gall-bladder; *B* liver; *C* adult bile. Gallbladder: bilirubin, taurodesoxycholic acid and traces of glycocholic and glycodesoxycholic acids are observed. Liver: bilirubin and an unidentified fraction are observed.

Moreover, we firmly believe that such cases of unstained meconium are also in favor of the hepatobiliary origin of the meconial bile. In fact, if the intestinal origin of bile is accepted and no pathology is found in the gut, a total reabsorption of the intestinal excretion would have to be involked. This never happens normally, as the meconium is always colored.

B. Conclusions

From the fact that physiologically, the meconial pigment is totally or predominantly a result of hepato-biliary secretion, it seems to be certain that: (1) *A normally colored meconium indicates that the pathological process,* biliary atresia or hepatitis, in its period of state, with a well-established cholestasis, *occurs after the time when the staining of the meconial matter takes place,* i.e. after the seventh or eighth month of intrauterine life, although the onset of the process could have taken place at a much earlier date. (2) Only in the cases where there is little or no staining of the meconium will the establishment of the period of stasis of the pathological process have to be dated to an earlier stage of pregnancy.

From these statements it follows that: In extrahepatic atresia, the frequent main sign (normal meconium) and the great chronological *disparity* between the pigmentation of the meconium and the organization of the excretory ducts make us reconsider and rectify the alledged developmental defect, the recanalization alteration, as its pathogenical determinism (p. 109).

The pathogenical theory of a recanalization defect, transmitted for years from one author to another, is not acceptable. We firmly believe that if a possible dysgenic influence is accepted as the etiology of extrahepatic atresia, it can mean no more than a greater susceptibility of the already present excretory ducts to the morbid agent that eventually will lead to destruction of the epithelium and later on to atresia.

Summary: A developmental disorder should be admitted, exclusively as secondary to a damage of the ducts. The partially or totally destroyed ducts obviously pose a difficulty or impossibility to a normal growth.

These two arguments: (1) the clinical sign of colored meconium, and (2) the pathological datum referred to in page 93, indicating that atresia results from a primary inflammatory process due to a cause that produces a lesion of the ducts, and is not secondary to their affection, *are the two main elements in the thesis that atresia is not a disontogenic process but an acquired one,* originated during postembryonic life. Further arguments in favor of this interpretation are given in the chapter that deals with etiology.

The rather frequent coincidence of two types of lesion, malformation and atresia, which is so difficult to understand to many authors, including, most recently, LILLY and STARZL [1974, chap. 1] can, in our opinion, be easily interpreted: these would be mixed cases, in which a blastoembryopathy (real malformation) is followed by a fetopathy producing atresia, or more simply, hepatitis.

B. Intrahepatic Atresia

The alledged obstruction of the large ducts by epithelial hyperplasia and the subsequent recanalization defect constitutes a very unlikely explanation of the pathogeny of atresia of the large bile ducts; but, could it account for the atresia of the small intrahepatic ones?

How can intrahepatic atresia, and especially the frequent mixed cases of extrahepatic and intrahepatic atresia be explained?

a) Ontogenical Defect

Some authors, like LANGMAN [1969], even tried to attribute intrahepatic atresia to a recanalization defect of the small ducts. The opinion of the majority of authors is at variance with this point of view. They admit a generation error. Can the point of view that intrahepatic atresia is really an agenesia be accepted?

Let us consider these problems in some detail:

Ontogenical defect of the intrahepatic bile ducts as the expression of a main malformation of the liver. Some authors [STOWENS, 1966, chap. 2] see in intrahepatic atresia, as in extrahepatic atresia, an embryological disorder corresponding to a primary malformation of the liver, presenting the following pathological features: distortion of the lobular architecture; absence or malformation of the ducts; rupture of trabecular architecture, and hyperplasia of branches of the hepatic artery leading to fibrosis, cirrhosis, massive irregular hyperplasia of the biliary epithelium, and bile stasis.

We believe the following arguments can be presented against this conception: (1) It is surprising that such a severe malformation of the liver parenchyma is not revealed in its external appearance. (2) The signs of malformation mentioned by STOWENS [1966, chap. 2] are not, in our opinion, exclusive of a developmental anomaly, as they can be observed in acquired inflammatory processes and their sequelae; a good number of authors [SILVERBERG, 1963; KISSANE and SMITH, 1967] object to the malformation of the liver admitted by STOWENS [1966, chap. 2]. (3) According to our observations, in cases of total extrahepatic and intrahepatic 'agenesia' (when there is minimal or no giant cell transformation), the lobular and trabecular architecture are essentially preserved, without signs of increase in the number or thickness of the arteries.

Ontogenical defect of the intrahepatic bile ducts as an expression of their own malformation. AHRENS *et al.* [1951, chap. 1] presented an important work on intrahepatic biliary atresia discussing their series of personal cases and reviewing a few other previously reported series, stressing the fact that both intrahepatic and extrahepatic atresia are *not* accompanied by malformation of the parenchyma. They admit an embryological disorder in the pathogeny of the intrahepatic atresia, which they explain as follows: 'New hepatic cells are formed from the primitive ones, whereas the development of the ducts is missing by virtue of yet unknown reasons.' This supposed dysontogeny is used by the authors to propose an embryological theory of the production of the bile ducts – that the hepatic parenchyma and the ducts form and grow independently, according to HAMMAR [1926]. An opposite view is held by AHRENS *et al.* as they consider that initially there is a single embryonic anlage for the parenchyma and the ducts.

As can be readily understood, the supposed dysembryogenic factor invoked to explain the pathogenesis of intrahepatic atresia would have to depart from the mechanism advocated by the theory[23] of channel formation.

b) Various Development Theories

Development of the external ducts. There are two conceptions to explain it: (1) they arise independently from a rudiment *of the cystic* anlage, and (2) they arise from an embryological anlage with elements that will originate other structures of the liver; parenchyma and internal ducts.

The first conception draws little support nowadays, in particular after it has been demonstrated that teratological agents, like thalidomide, which can produce an aplasia of the gallbladder, do *not* alter the remaining external ducts.

Development of the intrahepatic ducts. One of the various conceptions considers that the ducts, both internal and external, and the parenchyma are potentially contained in the hepatic primordium, and that their development with the subsequent differentiation of ducts and parenchyma is stimulated by the mesenchymal tissue of the septum transversum, acting as an inductor, according to the classical conception of this term. The fact that such mesenchymal connective tissue has an inductive action has been demonstrated in tissue culture studies by DOLJANSKY and ROULET [1934]. In cultures of liver and embryonic mesenchymal cells, these authors have found that the hepatic cells in contact with the mesenchyma form epithelium and lined cysts similar to bile ducts. Another fact to point out as evidence of the transforming activity of the connective tissue (even when it is beyond the mesenchymal stage), is the cholangiolar transformation of hepatic cells in postnecrotic cirrhosis, a phenomenon observed by POPPER and ELIAS [1955]. In this case, the plates of hepatic cells *(laminae hepatis)* develop into cholangial laminae, with two layers of cells and a lumen, while the appearance of the hepatic cells changes to look like a cubic epithelium; this occurs when the connective tissue proliferates in the spaces of Disse. This theory, proposed by BLOOM [1926], is currently accepted by many authors [AREY, 1946; HAMILTON *et al.*, 1962].

STREETER [1951] admits BLOOM's theory that parenchyma and ducts arise from the hepatic primordium and differentiate under the defining action of the mesenchyma, but maintains that the ducts originate from already constituted hepatic cells that grow from the center to the periphery. The first to form are the external ducts and later the internal ones, which will be of smaller size.

In another conception, a *totally independent origin for ducts and parenchyma*

---

23 The existence of several theories already suggests that none of them is unquestionably accurate.

is admitted; the intrahepatic ducts would develop from the extrahepatic ones to penetrate into the liver and reach the lobule [HAMMAR, 1926].

A mixed origin for the intrahepatic ducts, which would be partly ductal, partly parenchymal, has been proposed too. The larger intrahepatic ducts would result from the extrahepatic ones penetrating into the gland; while the small intrahepatic ones: (a) could be the result of the transformation of hepatic cells, becoming ducts, 'thanks to the mechanical influence' of the connective tissue, and later anastomosing with the larger penetrating ducts [HORTSMAN, 1962, chap. 2], or (b) could result from a 'recruitment' phenomenon, exerted by those larger ducts on the hepatic cells [ELIAS, 1967].

According to this author, a distinction must be established between 'recruitment' and 'induction'. By 'induction', we understand the action of one cell A upon antoher cell B, converting it into a C cell, different from both A and B. An example of induction is the influence of the notochord upon the primitive epidermis to transform it into the neural tube. Other examples would be the formation of all the bile excretory ducts, following BLOOM's theory, or that of the small intrahepatic ones, according to HORTSMAN's theory. In 'recruitment', one cell A acting upon another cell B transforms it into a cell of the A type.

c) None of the Mentioned Theories Can, on its own, Explain Dysontogenically the Pathogeny of the Different Types of Atresia – Extrahepatic, Intrahepatic or Mixed

1. The fact that in atresia there is always a normally patterned parenchyma, makes BLOOM's theory inapplicable to all types of atresia.

The ingenious dysembryogenical explanation given by STOWENS [1963] for the different types of atresia, based on a failure in the production of ducts following STREETER's theory[24], is not acceptable either, for the same reason that the malformation of the parenchyma that STOWENS [1963] invokes does not exist, as we have previously indicated (p. 129).

2. Intrahepatic atresia could be explained by HAMMAR's theory, admitting that the development of the ducts was interrupted once the external ones were formed. But such a theory is inapplicable to the case of isolated extrahepatic atresia, unless we accept that these external ducts are destroyed after being formed.

3. Considering HORTSMAN's statements, it is difficult to accept that a penetration defect of the external ducts should coincide with a failure in the inductive effect of the connective tissue, to explain total atresia; and, in any case, if such a possibility is accepted, this induction defect should

---

24   If the ontogenical disturbance occurs very early and does not persist, only the external ducts would fail to develop; if it occurs in a later period, only the internal ducts would be affected, and if the disorder persists for a long time, a mixed external and internal atresia would result.

be accompanied by a developmental disorder of the parenchyma. This does not occur, as has already been indicated, and ELÍAS' theory could explain intrahepatic atresia if it is accompanied by extrahepatic atresia, becuase in such a case the recruiters would be missing. But in isolated intrahepatic atresia, why would the recruiting action have failed? Would it not be more likely that the internal ducts did develop but were later destroyed? It is undeniable that even when the intrahepatic atresia is of the 'complete' or 'total' type, some remnants of those ducts can always be found, a fact that answers this question. How can the presence of normal intrahepatic ducts in isolated extrahepatic atresia be explained? To account for this fact in the frame of the propose theory, the destruction of the external ducts after having been organized would have to be admitted.

Summing up, the fact that one type of atresia can be explained by the failure of a determined form of development, but not the pathogeny of other types of atresia, would lead to admit several duct-generating mechanisms, a conclusion that seems to be *logically unacceptable*.

DANKS [1965, chap. 1] studied seven cases of intrahepatic atresia, and observed a progression of histological changes: from the initial appearance of large and irregularly proliferated bile ducts in the portal spaces to the complete absence of the small ones. Consequently, he indicates that: 'It seems probably that the small bile ducts have been destroyed more than even been constructed.'

We contend that this theory of DANKS, cautiously worded as 'it seems probable', should be more categorical and affirmative, as confirmed by the demonstration of a d-d-n process, which not only affects the proper excretory structures, but also those that result from the injury-reaction dynamics.

Conclusion: As the concept of a dysontogenetic mechanism to explain biliary atresia is unacceptable from the pathogenetical standpoint, we believe that such a process would have to be the result, at least in most cases, *not of a defective formation but of a deformation of already created ducts*.

C. Neonatal Hepatitis

The hypothesis linking the pathogeny of neonatal hepatitis with a developmental disorder has its most ardent defenders in SMETANA *et al.* [1965, chap. 2]. However, we believe that the arguments offered to support this hypothesis are of little weight (p. 146).

IV. Other Pathogenic Theories for the Entities of the Triad

A. For Both Extrahepatic and Intrahepatic Atresia-Disuse Atrophy

To consider that extrahepatic atresia constitutes an expression of a 'disuse atrophy' as some authors have suggested, is in our opinion quite unlikely at least as the main pathogenic cause. This is discussed with some detail when dealing with intrahepatic atresia (p. 156) for which such a pathogeny has been more specifically invoked.

B. For Extrahepatic Atresia-Ischemic Episode

Very recently, a new theory has been offered to explain extrahepatic atresia. PURI *et al.* [1974] contend that the findings in their cases indicate that an ischemia episode is a more likely event in the causation of extrahepatic atresia. This is born out by the fibrosis, the iron deposition in the fibrous tissue and the changes in the vessels which were seen in the duct remnants at the porta hepatis.

In our opinion, the epithelial lesions are usually so diffuse, although not evenly distributed, and the necrotic foci that appear to correspond to a lack of vascular supply so small that such a pathogeny as an exclusive explanation seems quite unlikely. The minor ischemic lesions that are indeed present could easily be accounted for by the common signs of thrombovasculitis found in all inflammatory processes.

References

ANDREWS, B. I.: Amniotic fluid study to determine maturity. Pediat. Clins N. Am. *17:* 49 (1970).

APODACA, J.; LANGE, W. und KOHLER, H.: Hepatitis bei Affen nach Verimpfung von Adenoviren aus Menschen mit Virus-Hepatitis. II. Histopathologische Befunde. Zentbl. Bakt. ParasitKde *207:* 100 (1968).

AREY, L. B.: Developmental anatomy, p. 226 (Saunders, Philadelphia 1946).

BETKE, K.: Bilirubin und Bilirubin-Ausscheidung; in LINNEWEH Die physiologische Entwicklung des Kindes, p. 172 (Springer, Berlin 1959).

BLANC, W. A.: cit. BRENT (chap. 1).

BLOOM, M.: Embryogenesis of human bile capillaries and ducts. Am. J. Anat. *36:* 451 (1926).

BÖHM: Ein Fall von kongenitaler Gallengangsatresie. Z. angew. Anat. Konstitutionslehre *1:* 105 (1913); cit. YLPPÖ (chap. 1).

BRODERSEN, R. and HERMANN, L. S.: Intestinal reabsorption of unconjugated bilirubin; a possible contributing factor in neonatal jaundice. Lancet *i:* 1242 (1962).

CARPENTER, H. M.: Pathogenesis of congenital jejunal atresia. Archs Path. *73:* 390 (1962).

CHERRY, S. H.: Amniotic fluid bilirubin as an index of fetal maturity. Am. J. Obstet. Gynec. *30:* 615 (1967).

COROMINAS-VILARDELL, A.: Unpublished data.

DOLJANSKY, L. und ROULET, F.: Über die gestaltende Wechselwirkung zwischen Epithel und Mesenchym. Virchows Arch. path. Anat. Physiol. *292:* 256 (1934); cit. ELIAS (chap. 5).

DUHAMEL, B.: Pathologie chirurgicale du nouveau-né et du nourrison; Spanish ed., p. 87 (Barcelona 1956).

DUHAMEL, B. et HAEGEL, P.: Malformations congénitales de l'intestin. Encycl. Med.-Chir. *9069A:* 10 (1964).

DUTTON, G. J.: Glucoronide synthesis in fetal liver and other tissues. Biochem. J. *71:* 141 (1959).

ELIAS, H.: Recruitment in human bile duct formation. Acta hepato-splenol. *14:* 253 (1967).

FASHENA, G. J.: Mechanism of hyperbilirubinaemia in the new-born infant. Am. J. Dis. Child. *76:* 146 (1948).

FINDLEY, L.; HIGGINS, G., and STAINER, M. H.: Icterus neonatorum: its incidence and cause. Archs Dis. Childh. *22:* 65 (1947).

FLEMING, A. and WOOLF, A. J.: Clin. chim. Acta *12:* 67 (1965); cit. WITH (chap. 1).

FRENSDORF: Ein Beitrag zur Kasuistik und Pathogenese der kongenitalen Gallengangsatresie. Frankf. Z. Path. *9:* 381 (1912); cit. YLPPÖ (chap. 1).

GARAY, E. R.; LOZZIO, B. B.; O'DONNEL, J. C.; TOCALINO, H. et EMILIANI, R.: Les pigments biliaires du méconium humain. Revue int. Hépat. *14:* 323 (1964).

GOHRBRANDT, E.; KARGER, P. und BERGMAN, E.: Chirurgische Krankheiten im Kindesalter; Spanish ed., p. 419 (Berlin 1928).

GROB, M.: Lehrbuch der Kinderchirurgie; Spanish ed., p. 429 (G. Thieme, Stuttgart 1957).

GUBERN-SALISACHS, L.: La maladie atrésiante des voies biliaires extrahépatiques. Archs fr. Pédiat. *25:* 415 (1968).

GUBERN-SALISACHS, L.: Personal commun. (1971).

HAI-CHIN-CHEN: Biliary cirrhosis related to prolonged obstructive neonatal jaundice. 11th Int. Congr. Ped., Tokyo 1965, p. 419.

HAMILTON, W. J.; BOYD, J. D., and MOSSMAN, H. W.: Human embryology, p. 241 (Heffer & Sons, Cambridge 1962).

HAMMAR, J. A.: Über die erste Entstehung der nicht-kapillaren intrahepatischen Gallengänge beim Menschen. Z. mikv. anat. Forsch. *5:* 59 (1926); cit. ELIAS.

HERINGOVÁ, A.; JIRSA, M., and JIRSOVA, V.: Biol. Neonate *6:* 277 (1964); cit. WITH (chap. 1).

HOLDER, T. M.: Atresia of extrahepatic bile duct. Am. J. Surg. *107:* 458 (1964).

HOLMES, A. W.; CAPPS, R. B., and DEINHARDT, R.: Results of inoculation of serum from patients with viral hepatitis into a subhuman primate. 9th Int. Congr. Microbiology, Moscow 1966, abstr., p. 394.

ISHIDA, M.; SAITO, F.; FAWAGUCHI, F.; NAKAJIO, T.; HANAWA, M.; TORIA, T., and SUCHIDA, K.: Surgical exploration in obstructive jaundice in infants. 11th Int. Congr. Pediat., Tokio 1965, p. 318.

JOHNSON, E. P.: The development of the mucous membrane of the oesophagous, stomac and small intestine in the human embryo. Am. J. Anat. *10:* 521 (1910).

KAYE, R.; WAGNER, B. M.; KOOP, C. E., and HOPE, J. W.: Needle biopsy of the liver and cholangiography as aids in the diagnosis of prolonged jaundice in infancy. Am. J. Dis. Child. *94:* 417 (1957).

KISSANE, J. M. and SMITH, M. G.: Pathology of infancy and childhood, pp. 291, 293 (C. V. Mosby, St. Louis 1967).

KLEINSCHMIDT, H.: Angeborener Verschluss und Stenose des Dünn- und Dickdarms; in PFAUNDLER und SCHLOSSMANN Handbuch der Kinderheilkunde, p. 283 (Vogel Verlag, Berlin 1931).

KO, V.; DUTTON, G. J., and NEMETH, A. M.: Development of uridine diphosphate glucoronyltransferase activity in cultures of chick-embryo liver. Biochem. J. *104:* 991 (1967).

KÖHLER, H. und APODACA, J.: Hepatitis bei Affen nach Verimpfung von Adenoviren aus Menschen mit Virushepatitis. I. Bestimmung der Enzymaktivitäten im Verlauf der Erkrankung. Zentbl. Bakt. Infekt. Hyg. *206:* 1 (1968).

KREUTER: cit. KLEINSCHMIDT.

KÜNZER, W.; WAHLENKAMP, H. und FÖSTER, B.: Zur Frage einer direkten Bilirubinpassage aus dem Blut ins Darmlumen. Beobachtungen an Kindern mit angeborener Gallengangatresie oder Darmatresie. Dt. med. Wschr. *90:* 2096 (1965).

LANDING, B. H.: Considerations of the pathogenesis of neonatal hepatitis, biliary atresia and choledocal cyst. The concept of infantile obstructive cholangiopathy. Acquisitions en chirurgie infantile, tome 6, p. 113 (Masson et Cie, Paris 1974).

LANGMAN, J.: Medical embryology; Spanish ed., pp. 236, 237 (Williams & Wilkins, Baltimore 1969).

LARSEN, E. H. and WITH, T. K.: Chemical, biological and clinical aspects; in WITH Bile Pigments, p. 592 (Academic Press, New York 1948).

LAURITZEN, C. and LEHMANN, W.: The significance of steroid hormones for the development of hyperbilirubinaemia and icterus in the newborn infant. J. Endocr. *39:* 183 (1967).

LEREBOULLET, N.: cit. DUHAMEL.

LESTER, R.; BERHRMAN, R. E., and LUCEY, J. F.: Transfer of bilirubin C-14 across monkey placenta. Pediatrics, Springfield *32:* 416 (1963).

LESTER, R. and SCHMID, R.: Intestinal absorption of bile pigments. New Engl. J. Med. *264:* 178 (1963).

MACKAY, E. V. and WATSON, D.: The prognostic values of bilirubin levels in amniotic fluid in rhesus iso-immunized pregnancies. Med. J. Aust. *49:* 942 (1962).

MANDELBAUM, B.; LACROIX, G. C., and ROBINSON, A. R.: Determination of fetal maturity by spectrophotometric analysis of amniotic fluid. Am. J. Obstet. Gynec. *29:* 471 (1967).

MAYNADIER, A.; GUILLAUD, R.; BARRET, Cl.; POUS, J. G. et ADREY, J.: Péritonites biliaires néonatales, formes calcifiantes et formes nécrosantes. Com. Session Annu. Soc. Française Pédiatrie, Montpellier 1970.

MOUTSOURIS, C.: The 'solid stage' and congenital intestinal atresia. J. pediat. Surg. *1:* 446 (1967).

OBERNIEDERMAYER, A.: Lehrbuch der Chirurgie und Orthopädie des Kindesalters; vol. 2, part II, pp. 211, 339 (Springer, Berlin 1959).

OSKI, F. A. and NAIMAN, J. F.: Hematologic problems in the newborn, p. 144 (Saunders, Philadelphia 1966).

PETERMAN, M. G.: Neonatal hepatitis in siblings. J. Pediat. 50: 315 (1953).

PICKETT, L. K.: in BENSON, MUSTARD, RAVITCH, SNYDER and WELCH Pediatric surgery, p. 620 (Year Book Med. Publishers, Chicago 1962).

POLAND, R. L. and ODELL, G. B.: Physiological jaundice. The enterohepatic circulation of bilirubin. New Engl. J. Med. 284: 1 (1971).

POPPER, H. and ELIAS, H.: Histogenesis of hepatic cirrhosis studied by the three-dimensional approach. Am. J. Path. 31: 405 (1955).

PORTER, S. D.; SOPER, R. T., and TIDRICK, R. T.: Biliary hypoplasia. Ann. Surg. 177: 602 (1968).

PURI, P.; CARROLL, R.; O'DONNELL, J., and QUINEY, E. J.: A view on the actiology of extrahepatic biliary atresia. 21st Int. Congr. Br. Ass. Paediat. Surgeons, Bern 1974, abstr., p. 36.

RAPOPORT, M.: in MITCHELL-NELSON Text book of pediatrics; Spanish ed., p. 1318 (Saunders, Philadelphia 1950).

RAPOPORT, M.: in NELSON Text book of pediatrics, p. 704 (Saunders, Philadelphia 1959).

REHBEIN, F. und NEUMANN, G.: Angeborene Gallengangsatresie. Kinderärztl. Praxis 26: 78 (1957).

RIETZ, T.: Über die normale und abnormale Entwicklung der extrahepatischen Gallenwege. Nord. med. Akad. 50: 1 (1917); cit. in ARANDES, BALLESTER y ALCALDE Afecciones de la vía biliar principal, p. 244 (Ed. JIMS, Barcelona 1963).

ROLLESTON, H. D. and HAYENDE, L. B.: Case of congenital hepatic cirrhosis with oliterative cholangitis (congenital obliteration of the bile ducts). Br. med. J. i: 758 (1901); cit. STRAUSS and BERNSTEIN (chap. 3).

ROSA, P.: Etude de la circulation du liquide amniotique humain. Gynéc. Obstét. 50: 463 (1951).

ROSTA, J.; MAKOI, Z., and KERTESZ, A.: The role of delayed meconium passage in neonatal hyperbilirubinaemia, 12th Int. Congr. Pediat., Mexico 1968, vol. 3, p. 655.

ROUVIÈRE, H.: cit. DUHAMEL.

SHENKER, S.; BAWBER, N. H., and SCHMID, R.: Bilirubin metabolism in the fetus. J. clin. Invest. 43: 32 (1964).

SCHMID, R. and HAMMAKER, L.: Trans. Ass. Am. Physns 75: 220 (1962); cit. KÜNZER, WAHLENKAMP and FÖSTER.

SCHRIEDE: cit. KLEINSCHMIDT.

SHIRKEY, H. C.: Pediatric therapy (St. Louis 1964); cit. KÜNZER, WAHLENKAMP and FÖSTER.

SILVERBERG, M.: In discussion to paper of D. STOWENS.

SMITH, D. W.: Recognizable patterns of human malformation, last page (Saunders, Philadelphia 1970).

STOWENS, D.: Congenital biliary atresia. Ann. N.Y. Acad. Sci. 111: 337 (1963).

STRANSKY, E. and LARA, R. T.: On neonatal hepatitis and its sequelae. Simultaneously a report on a case of congenital atresia of the bile ducts combined with infectious hepatitis with giant cell formation. Annls paediat. *195:* 145 (1960).

STREETER, G. L.: Developmental horizons in human embryos (Carnegie Institution, Washington 1951); cit. STOWENS (chap. 1).

TESTUT, L. y LATARJET, A.: Tratado de anatomía humana, vol. 4, p. 354 (Salvat, Barcelona 1944).

TANDLER, J.: Gegenbauers Morph. Jb. *29:* 62 (1902); cit. KÜNZER, WAHLENKAMP and FÖSTER.

TER-GRIGOROWA, H.: Fetale und neonatale Hepatitiden und deren Folgen. Zentbl. allg. Path. path. Anat. *108:* 297 (1965).

THOMPSON, J.: Edib. med. J. *37:* 523, 604, 724, 1112 (1891–92); cit. AHRENS *et al.* (chap. 1) and SWEET (chap. 2).

VÉGHELY, P. V.: Stoffwechsel, Ernährung, Verdauung; in OPITZ und SCHMID Handbuch der Kinderheilkunde, Spanish ed., vol. 4, p. 1299 (Springer, Berlin 1964).

VEST, M.: Physiologie und Pathologie des Neugeborenenikterus. Biblthca paediat., No. 69, p. 46 (Karger, Basel 1959).

YLPPÖ, A.: Icterus Neonatorum (ind. I. n. gravis) und Gallenfarbstoffsekretion beim Fötus und Neugeborenen. Z. Kinderheilk. *9:* 218 (1913a).

ZWEIFEL: Arch. Gynaek. *7:* 474 (1875); cit. YLPPÖ and BETKE.

Chapter 6

Etiology of the Entities of the Triad

Having pointed out the common pathogenical determinism of the triad, the idea of a correspondence between a pathogenical and an etiological unit is, at least, very suggestive. Consequently, few authors argue against the likelihood of this idea, proposed as a work hypothesis by ALAGILLE [1965, chap. 1] and recently described by PILLOUD [1966, chap. 1] as follows: 'Hepatitis virus could be responsible for neonatal hepatitis, intrahepatic agenesias, and extrahepatic atresia according to the respectively late or more or less precocious affectation of the fetal liver and the degree of development of the biliary embryonic rudiments at that moment.' We agree with this hypothesis suggesting: (1) to change the expression 'intrahepatic agenesia' by that of 'atresia', and the 'one of more or less precocious' by that of 'less or more', and (2) we do not consider as a so decissive a factor the precocity of involvement of the liver, an element that would determine, according to PILLOUD the likelihood of involvement of the large ducts.

The hepatitis virus, we equally believe, should be held responsible for the great majority of cases and maybe with some differences in pathology between the viruses A and B. The etiological theories ascribed to each one of the entities of the triad will now be separately reviewed.

I. Extrahepatic Atresia

A. Genetic Cause (Dysgenia)
This is due to a disturbance of the genic material, the 'germinal plasma'.

1. As an Expression of a Hereditary Pathological Manifestation

a) Dominant type of inheritance. The data we possess are totally against this form of inheritance.

b) Recessive type of inheritance. The familial character of some observations could suggest this etiology. Some of these observations are: (a) old, sure, proven cases, like those of GOULD [1855], BING [1866], YLPPÖ [1913, chap. 1], and SIMMEL [1921–22]; or only probable ones, like those of GLAISTER [1879], and THOMAS [1891]; (b) among the *more recent* cases (within the last 40 years), some are solidly proven ones, like those of SWEET [1932, chap. 2], HOPKINS [1941], WHITTEN and ADIE [1952], RUMLER [1961, chap. 1], KRAUS [1964], and NEGRO and LARGUERO [1965, chap. 3]. But in comparison to the large number of isolated observations, their number is so small that even admitting a small penetration of the pathological gene, it is very difficult to accept such a method of transmission, so that if we take the term 'familial' as an expression of an inherited genetic anomaly, such observations would really be only pseudofamilial.

The presence of other affected persons among the ancestors has only been pointed out exceptionally, as the reference to an avuncular uncle, in three familial cases, by RUMLER [1961, chap. 1]; but no unquestionable pathological proof of the diagnosis could be obtained. In fact, the expression 'without family history' constitutes the stereotype in each case of atresia. Finally, the fact of *consanguinity*, another common feature in the recessive hereditary traits, has not been found in atresia, but it has been reported in hepatitis, according to DANKS and BODIAN [1963, chap. 1].

2. Mutational

Can an anomaly of the germinal plasma occur by genic mutation?

It is well known that certain organic and functional diseases may be due to a mutational genic alteration, which can later be hereditarily transmitted, sometimes as a dominant trait; the mutational cases appear to be more frequent than the inherited ones. This is what occurs, e.g. with hemophilia vera, in which, according to QUICK [1960], only one fifth of the cases are the result of hereditary transmission, with known cases in their kinship, while the other four fifths are mutational. Something similar occurs in ataxia telangiectasia, with more than half the cases also of a mutational nature [PÉREZ-SOLER and ESPADALER, 1964].

In the present state of our knowledge, the mutational-genetical etiology of extrahepatic biliary atresia cannot be categorically denied, but cannot be confirmed either. We will have a definite verdict on the possibility of such a mutation, knowing that every mutational factor is hereditarily transmitted, in the discovery of cases with members in their progeny affected by biliary atresia who have been cured. Up to now, as far as we know, no cases of this nature have been reported. In our judgment, nevertheless, we believe that if such cases are possible, they will have to be exceptional, because our observations and thinking have led us to admit that such a disease should be attributed in the great majority of cases, if not in all, to an acquired noxa acting past the organogenic period.

3. Presence of Cases of Atresia in Diseases Due to Inherited Functional Anomalies of Genes and in Processes Dependent on Chromosomal Alterations (Anomalies in Number or Structure of Chromosomes)

Biliary atresia has been exceptionally described in some cases of pancreatic cystic fibrosis [in a recent report by PERALTA et al., 1968]. So far, no anomalies in the number and structure of the chromosomes have been described in biliary atresia. It is surprising and worth special mention that in cases of chromosomal aberrations, even with a marked polymorphism of the defects observed, biliary atresia has very rarely been found. This is what occurs, for example, with mongolism.

In WOLF's [1964] monography in which the semiology of Down's syndrome is gathered with great detail, among the 134 cases considered there is not a single instance of biliary atresia. Nevertheless, this concomitance has been pointed out in two cases reported by DANKS and CAMPBELL [1966, chap. 2].

At present, the etiology of these very rare observations of biliary atresia associated with illnesses with a functional or anatomical disturbance of the genic material cannot be satisfactorily accounted for. The small number of reported cases does not permit a statistical evaluation.

However, it may be logically assumed that: (1) they might correspond to a rare manifestation of these dysgenical entities, although this seems unlikely; (2) they can merely result from a chance association, or (3) perhaps they could be explained by the greater susceptibility of congenitally malformed individuals to other pathological agents. In relation to this, we may quote the above-mentioned cases of mongolism: they clearly constitute a case of chromosomal aberration, resulting in a great variety of malformations and an extraordinary propensity from an early age in extrauterine life to infectious processes, especially affecting the respiratory tract.

In relation to the concomitance of biliary atresia and other malformative processes due to chromosomal aberrations, it is worth mentioning the relation with trisomy 18 [WINDMILLER et al., 1965; WEICHSEL and

LUZZATTI, 1965]. Surprisingly, the association of neonatal hepatitis with it has also been reported [initial case of EDWARDS *et al.*, 1960], as are other processes of a malformative or inflammatory kind, such as hypoplasia of the extrahepatic ducts [case of SMITH *et al.*, 1962] fibrocystic liver [case of BUTLER *et al.*, 1965] or jaundice with round cell infiltration of the liver [case of GERMAN, 1962]. These possibilities of pathological symbiosis have recently been confirmed by ALPERT *et al.* [1969]: In a group of 10 cases of trisomy 18 proven by cytogenetic studies, signs of hepatitis were found in 3 of them; of 9 cases with the phenotypic features of the syndrome (without cytogenetic study), 4 presented similar hepatic lesions, and in 2 of them there was evidence of extrahepatic atresia.

Concerning this possible relationship between the trisomy 18 syndrome and the entities of the triad, two other points still deserve special mention:

1. In a series of 60 cases of this chromosomal aberration collected from the literature, only 6 (already referred to) showed a concomitance of the dysmorphic syndrome with the hepatic injury described. But recently, ALPERT *et al.* [1969] reported 7 such associations in 19 cases of trisomy. The great difference between these figures will reasonably lead one to search for an *added cause* in ALPERT's series which could explain the common occurrence of hepatitis or of hepatitis with extrahepatic atresia among their cases. Statistical analysis of these figures suggests that the probabilities of existence of one such cause are great ($0.01 < p < 0.05$).

2. The presentation of mixed cases of hepatitis and atresia constitute in our opinion evidence that: (a) both must be *intimately related* from a *pathogenic point of view* – in all likelihood, as the expression of a destructive inflammatory process, and (b) from an *etiological point of view*, if they are not the result of a single agent, it should be admitted that both producing causes, in virtue of a very exceptional circumstance, have coincided in a syndrome which is quite infrequent.

B. Acquired Cause
1. During the Blasto-Embryonic Period

Considering the high incidence of congenital or innate malformations of a postconceptionally acquired etiology, usually during embryonic life, a certain number of authors have very recently tended to admit the existence of a noxa acting during the organogenic period:

STOWENS [1959, chap. 1] talks of an unknown environmental agent which would act traumatizing the ducts and preventing the transformation of the hepatic cells into ducts, according to STREETER's embryological conception.

None of the toxic agents known by their teratological value (iodine, selenium, etc.) seem to be responsible. Even the last entry in the list, thalidomide, which is known to be capable of producing an aplasia of the gallbladder and on a few occasions a stenosis of the bile duct [KAJÜ, 1965], must be discarded as in no case thalidomide figured in the antecedents.

The viral agents have been – since GREGG [1941] – found very often responsible for many malformations; it is quite understandable that the idea of a viral etiology has been suggested by many authors.

Special attention has been devoted to the *hepatitis virus*, as we are dealing with an hepatopathy which usually has not other significant extrahepatic pathological manifestations, though a fair number of cases is associatet with malformations, as has been mentioned. This virus is known to be the most hepatopathic; other viruses, such as the mononucleosis virus, are very much less hepatopathic in their action. Also, the Coxsackie virus, according to recent contributions, has a hepatopathic role, which is considered more important every day [BLATNER, 1966]. This would suggest that virological studies will have to be necessarily carried out while searching for an etiological diagnosis of the triad, and a special consideration must be given to the possible role which this enterovirus can play.

It is true that this viral hepatitic etiology has been always proposed with great diffidence, more as a possibility than as a probability, sometimes only proposed as a working hypothesis: (1) because the epidemiological relation of cases of atresia with such a virus is very obscure, and seemingly nonexistent; (2) because at the present moment there is no biological, serological or cutaneous hypersensitivity test, to demonstrate with certainty that a disease recognizes the hepatitis virus as a causal agent, and (3) because the demonstration of a viral agent, specifically the transmission to an experimental animal, has not been possible up to a very recent date. HOLMES *et al.* [1966, chap. 5] have managed to reproduce viral hepatitis in the South American marmoset monkey *(Sanguinus oedipus)* producing a disease very similar, if not identical, to that observed in the human species. This work has been confirmed by KÖHLER and APODACA [1968, chap. 5] and APODACA *et al.* [1968, chap. 5], who have found the same enzymatic and pathological alterations pointed out by the mentioned American authors. This technique for detecting the virus as the supposed etiological agent has not yet been applied to the field of the triad, or at least no reports have appeared so far in the literature.

It is certain, of course, that *a virus acting during the embryonic period is not clearly seen,* though we must have in mind the two following points:

1. Extrahepatic biliary atresia was not mentioned among the multiple malformations characterizing rubella embryopathy. Nevertheless, neonatal hepatitis has been recently reported as a contingency of antenatal rubella, with the malformative tetrad characteristic and typical of this viric embryopathy (see below and p. 164) and even with giant cell transformation, but it seems [ESTERLY *et al.,* 1967, chap. 3] without ductal lesions although with ductular proliferation. Up to a very recent date [STRAUSS and BERNSTEIN, 1968, chap. 3], no case of atresia that could be attributed to the rubella virus had been described. *Nevertheless, the fact of its being accompanied by other malformations does not necessarily prove that such an atresia must be of embryonic origin* (see below).

2. The observations of EMMERT [1969] have significantly pointed out that the *hepatitis virus only produces unspecific lesions in the embryo,* very similar to those produced by the rubella and the parotiditis virus. These viruses *cause only minimal or no hepatic lesions:* they produce a very characteristical embryopathic syndrome, which TÖNDURY [1965] classifies as a viral embryopathic syndrome with 'selective' effect on the brain, the vascular system (heart), the lens in the eye and the ear, as paramount manifestations. Such a group of 'selective' embryopathic malformations are certainly not an accompanying feature either of atresia or of hepatitis, *but very often some developmental defects are seen in these entities* (pp. 120 ff.).

Thus, the embryopathological studies of EMMERT [1969] offer a basis to assert the teratogenic action of the hepatitis virus on the embryo; but it should be emphasized that *this action is not exerted upon the liver or the bile ducts.*

Usually, and unlike what occurs with rubella, the embryo survives this malformation syndrome with difficulty. This is how the facts should be logically explained: (1) After the investigations of EMMERT [1969], carried out in embryos obtained from therapeutic abortions which were processed immediately after being obtained, thus providing for study suitable material, free of the necrobiotic component customarily found in specimens obtained from spontaneous abortion, and (2) the review by THALHAMMER [1967] of several papers (table VI), uncovering the fact that 25% of the pregnancies in women who suffered a viral hepatitis during the first three months of pregnancy are miscarried, it seems that only very few cases are spared from this severe embryonic teratogenic action, resulting in diverse malformations. DORFLER'S [1957] paper gives a perfect idea of the rarity of such cases: he found in his extensive review of the literature only 15 cases of malformations that could be attributed to the hepatitis virus. However, our concept is that if one adds to these cases those which later on develop an icteric syndrome due to hepatitis or atresia, the number of cases would become considerably larger.

2. During the Fetal Period

On considering this problem, the following basic facts must be mentioned:

1. Although perhaps in some cases they may be possible, the embryonic etiologies have been discarded.

2. The presence of meconium, generally with normal characteristics, patently shows that the liver had been functioning when the cholestasis began.

3. The process is of an inflammatory nature (this being a sign of fetopathy rather than embryopathy, as is already well known, and as TÖNDURY [1965] has once more confirmed in his studies), and we have already reasoned about its primary, determining character in atresia (p. 93) showing it is not a secondary event of atresia.

4. The presence of differentiated morphological elements, especially epithelial crypts and muscular fiber bundles, doubtlessly certifies that there had been an organized structure.

This means that the bile ducts have been injured already in full postorganogeic period; the noxa must have carried out its deleterious action on them during the fetal period, although it can be admitted that the morbid influence might have begun earlier in full embryonic period, in the cases where atresia is accompanied by malformations of other organs.

Now, before further speculating on the etiology of extrahepatic atresia (p. 144), it is in order to consider why such a destructive process of the bile ducts takes place during the fetal-perinatal period.

It is certain that injuries of a similar type, with the exception of those due to a traumatic or neoplasic cause (circumstances which arise only exceptionally during fetal life) do not frequently occur in extrauterine life. In particular, atresia of the large external ducts of a *primary* kind, *not secondary* to trauma, neoplasia, etc., seems to be exceptional in the adult and also in the child.

How can this *obliteration of the extrahepatic ducts* be explained? By approaching the general problem of susceptibility of a given individual to the various pathologies. Considering what has been said, it appears that this must basically be a question of disposition to a given type of pathology in which, as is well known, two types of factors must be taken into account: the predominantly *endogenous* and the predominantly *exogenous*.

a) Predominantly Endogenous Factors

These are, as is well known, age, sex, race, etc.

Age is the main factor and the only one to be dealt with. Its importance was stressed when pointing out that the younger the person the greater the possibility of destruction of his hepatic excretory ducts. It is now important to define whether this susceptibility is related to a *quantitative* or to a *qualitative* aspect of the ducts, i.e. whether they are more vulnerable because they are of a smaller size, short and with a very narrow lumen, or because some intrinsic conditions make the epithelial element more vulnerable.

We believe that both aspects play a role:

a) The smaller ducts: the external ones, with the appearance of an epithelial tube with a slightly furrowed lining and with sparse supporting structures – very thin middle and external layers at this early age – and the intrahepatic ones constituted by mere tubes, appear quite logically to be more susceptible to damage than others of a larger size; it would seem that this point requires no further elaboration.

b) The higher vulnerability of the epithelium is discussed in the following paragraphs.

It is a general law that the immunobiological response of a cell to a noxious agent, which may at times be refractory or show a hightened susceptibility, is closely related to its degree of anatomical and, especially, of functional differentiation; the type of response of the cells in these cases is not totally defined until they become mature. This helps to explain some immunological behavior which could seem paradoxical, if not absurd.

The behavior of the liver against the hepatitis virus may be taken as a good example.

During the embryonic period, both the hepatocyte and the cells of the excretory ducts are refractory to the hepatitis virus, as the studies of TÖNDURY [1965] and EMMERT [1969] have pointed out with precision. In extrauterine life, once the organ has reached maturity, the hepatocyte becomes the most susceptible epithelial element, its response to the viral attack varying from a lesion of the cellular membrane up to the necrosis of the cell, with a subsequent enzyme liberation. A logical following to this observed fact is to admit that in the period of semimaturity[25], throughout the fetal life, the hepatocyte and the cell of the excretory ducts will be in a state of intermediate immunity, meaning that the ductal cells will show a certain susceptibility to the virus, or that they may even exhibit an increased susceptibility during this period. This is our conception which is summarized in table V.

25 Semimaturity of the hepatocyte, quite obviously extended into the neonatal period, in certain aspects, as in glucoronyltransferase deficiency.

Table V. Morbid effect of the hepatitis virus on the hepatic parenchyma and excretory ducts

| | Intrauterine period | | Extrauterine period |
	embryo	fetus	
Anatomical and functional state of the liver	immaturity	semimaturity	maturity
Viral action	nonspecific	more specific	specific
Injury on:			
Hepatocyte	none	some	marked
Bile duct	none	some (probably marked)	slight

b) Predominantly Exogenous Factors

This category applies to the responsible agent, environmental factors, etc.

Only the agent will be dealt with.

Could it be that the hepatopathic agent (which is truly hepatopathic as, from a clinical and analytic point of view, its deleterious action is limited to the liver) would show a definite tendency to primarily harm the excretory system? We believe it is possible, but difficult to demonstrate in the present state of our theoretical-scientific knowledge.

5. Since the atresia-inducing agent acts in most cases well into the fetal period, as previously noted, and taking into account the dominant, if not specific, hepatopathic character of the agent, the focus of research should be logically directed to the *hepatitis virus as the most likely cause.*

Certainly, no case of atresia has shown clinical or analytic signs pointing to other diseases as the responsible agents. Thus, in no case has it been possible to incriminate any of the following etiological agents:

1. *Infections* due to banal bacterial flora, parasites (toxoplasma, treponema, etc.), other viruses (parotiditis, mononucleosis, herpes, echo, Coxsakie[26], etc.).

2. *Metabolic errors* – pancreatic cystic fibrosis, galactosemia, ornithinemia.

HARRIS [1965, chap. 2] and ANDERSEN [chap. 3] suggested that the ducts epithelium can be damaged by an abnormal bile. A primary metabolical disorder of such a nature has not been demonstrated, although obviously the bile produced by a diseased organ probably will differ from normal bile and perhaps have a deleterious

26   It has been recently pointed out by STRAUSS and BERNSTEIN [1968, chap. 3] that it is to be accepted that the rubella virus can cause atresia. For further information, see page 175.

effect on the excretory structures. Experimental confirmation of this possibility
(p. 73) may be offered by the reported observation that simple ductal ligation causes lesions in the parenchyma and excretory ducts, although the latter are initially of
a proliferative type.

3. *Drugs and toxic agents* – these factors are, it seems, always missing.

4. *Disuse,* which could be a cause of hypotrophy, dystrophy, especially in the
postnatal period, and has been considered a causal element in extrahepatic atresia
(this point is further considered when discussing etiology of intrahepatic atresia,
p. 156).

The exclusion of other agents, therefore, paves the way to the concept that the hepatitis virus is the responsible agent, its pathological action being carried out during the fetal period.

Nevertheless, in very few cases the hepatitis virus appears to be the producing
agent: these cases are limited to those of pathological and clinical interrelation between atresia and neonatal hepatitis (pp. 58, 103) and to those where the mother is
known to have suffered a viral hepatitis during pregnancy or the newborn presents
it. As BRENT [1962, chap. 1] points out, when the relative frequency of neonatal
hepatitis of viral origin is considered, the cases of atresia with a possible etiological
vinculation with the hepatitis virus are exceptional. Only on one occasion has the
hepatitis virus been found in a case of atresia [COLE *et al.*, 1965], although it had
been investigated only in three cases. In summary, it would seem that the relationship between the hepatitis virus and the production of atresia would merely be a
matter of chance.

We believe that the answer to two negative aspects which up to now
had been considered as very important in discussing or even rejecting
such an etiology constitute very valuable arguments at least for admitting
that the hepatitis virus is one of the producing agents: (1) The fact that a
case of atresia can rarely be related to a present or past hepatic viral disease of the mother, and (2) affected mothers only exceptionally give birth
to children with atresia. We believe it is easy to answer these arguments
following the general rules of epidemiology and the peculiar pathology of
the hepatitis virus. However, as these two negative aspects are also present in neonatal hepatitis, although not in such a conclusive way, we refer
the reader to section II C.

II. Neonatal Hepatitis

The usual and obvious inflammatory appearance of this process led
the earlier authors describing giant cell hepatitis to accept an infectious
etiology.

A. Infectious Etiology

CRAIG and LANDING [1952, chap. 2], BODIAN and NEWNS [1953], DIBLE *et al.* [1954, chap. 3] and others invoke an infectious process presumably of viral origin, and perhaps related to epidemic hepatitis or due to homologous serum disease and acquired *in utero* by transplacental transmission.

Trying to be more specific, some authors [STOCKES *et al.*, 1951, 1954; FRISELL and LUNDQUIST, 1955; ROTH and DUNCAN, 1955; GAL, 1956–57] held both viruses responsible. A majority [JANNEWAY, 1951; BODIAN and NEWNS, 1953; GELLIS, 1954; SCOTT *et al.*, 1954, chap. 2; CLAIREAUX, 1960; SHERLOCK, 1963, chap. 1] admit only as responsible the virus of homologous serum hepatitis, arguing that the viremia due to epidemic hepatitis is short-lasted and gives rise to the production of antibodies which would protect the fetus from the effect of the virus.

This explanation was given by JANNEWAY in 1951 and is repeatedly quoted by the authors. The B virus, on the other hand, produces a viremia of longer duration than the A virus, and this fact would explain the existence of familial cases (which would be in fact pseudofamilial cases).

The viral etiology was apparently proven by STOCKES *et al.* [1951] in an isolated case. Other authors, also attempting to transmit the disease to volunteers by injecting them with blood of the mother and the child failed to duplicate STOCKES' results. Recently, COLE *et al.* [1965], have managed to demonstrate by culture the presence of hepatitis virus in the three cases of neonatal hepatitis they investigated. The number of observations is undoubtedly small to reach a final decision, but it does permit to argue that the hepatitis virus is at least one of the possible agents. On this subject an unrestricted statement is not allowed unless the classical Koch's postulates are fulfilled: (1) the agent should be found in all cases of the disease we are concerned with; (2) this agent should not be found in any other disease as a casual and not morbid parasite, and (3) it should be completely isolated from the body and succesfully grown in a culture medium from where it could be transmitted to experimental animals.

Obviously, a full demonstration of the etiological role of the hepatitis virus fulfilling Koch's postulates has not been achieved, although many arguments for defending do exist; they will be further discussed in section II.C. Unquestionably, other possible etiologies could be assumed or argued for.

B. Other Incriminated Etiologies
1. Dysgenic, Due to an Alteration of the Germinal Plasma
1. Of a *definite* nature, expressed as a recessive hereditary manifestation. Let us discuss the elements which are offered in favor of this hereditary.

HSIA *et al.* [1958] and especially DANKS and BODIAN [1963, chap. 1] have suggested this way of transmission (with the consubstantial genic alteration) based on the fact that the number of those affected is close to the figure that corresponds to such a type of inheritance (0.250), and they point out at the same time that the process would be essentially due to a metabolical disorder, although the action of a virus (!) would constitute the determining element of the disease.

Several objections can be opposed to this conception of the recessive inheritance as THALHAMMER [1967] has pointed out: (1) The figures given by DANKS and BODIAN [1963, chap. 1] of the total of people affected, even accepting some doubtful cases, reaches only 0.141 ± 0.038, i.e. a figure clearly inferior to the one established as characteristic for such an inheritance. One could perhaps admit a smaller penetration of the pathological gene, but the figures given by GELLIS *et al.* [1954, chap. 1], who in a study of the families of 41 patients find only one familial case, are even lower. (2) In the extensive review of the literature on familial cases gathered up by THALHAMMER [1967], he is surprised by the fact that in a sibship where two or more cases occur, they are never mixed with normal sibs. In fact, they will appear in succession, one following the other. (3) THALHAMMER [1967] also points out that the cases that precede and follow the patient are not regularly distributed either: both in DANKS and BODIAN's [1963, chap. 1] as in GELLIS *et al.*'s [1954, chap. 1] series, the first are, by far, the predominant ones.

More arguments still cast serious doubt, if not completely reject, the recessive inheritance as a dysgenical etiology of neonatal hepatitis:

a) Consanguinity, another relevant factor when considering inheritance, has been pointed out in neonatal hepatitis [DANKS and BODIAN, 1963, chap. 1] and not in atresia; but the small figures (4 out of 45 families) apparently have not allowed a statistical evaluation.

Nevertheless, as is well known, consanguinity expresses not only the determinism of the propagation of a pathological gene, but also the simple disposition to suffer the effect of an acquired noxa: toxic, infections or other.

b) The study of the progeny and kinship does not provide positive information favoring a recessive inheritance which is held responsible for neonatal hepatitis.

In a study of the progeny in 45 families with cases of neonatal hepatitis carried out by DANKS and BODIAN [1963, chap. 1], which included 310 uncles and aunts and 469 first cousins, *no* suspicious case of neonatal hepatitis was uncovered.

c) Finally, the study of twins not only does not contribute any element in favor of the dysgenic theory, but according to our theory, does the opposite.

According to our information, up to 1966 the reported cases of neonatal hepatitis in twins were as follows: 6 cases in dizygotic twins in which only one member of each pair was clinically ill and jaundiced[27]; 2 cases in homozygotic twins of which in one both sibs were affected and in the other only one of them[28], and 1 case in unclassified twins with both sibs affected[29].

The presentation of the disease in both individuals of a pair of monozygotic twins and in only one in each pair of dizygotic ones corresponds to the manifestation of an inherited genetic character, according to the classical conception of heredity in twins. However, how can we explain the fact that only one was affected in another pair of monozygotic twins? If in this pair only one is affected, or shows a susceptibility to the disease in an unapparent, subclinical fashion, without jaundice, it must be accepted that hepatitis constitutes a sign which is not included in the constellation of common characters of the monozygotes, which may be a plausible argument. In both circumstances, of course, it would correspond to a very small susceptibility (only about 2–3% of cases f fetal neonatal hepatitis are due to epidemic hepatitis transmitted by the mother, p. 151). This easily explains that even when the fetus suffers the attack of the morbid noxa he is not affected by it, at least in a clincally ostensible fashion. Thus, of the 6 pairs of dizygotic twins which are known, only one in each pair would have suffered the disease, and the nonaffectation of the remaining cases would therefore probably have nothing to do with recessive inheritance.

2. Of an *undetermined* nature. The frequent presence of a great number of giant cells in hepatitis and in a good number of cases of atresia, has

---

27 MILLERS's [1957] case, with a no histological diagnosis of neonatal hepatitis with giant cells; three of LELONG et al.'s [1960, 1961] cases with a proved diagnosis; one of WONG et al.'s [1965] cases with a proved diagnosis; one of PILLOUD's [1966b, chap. 1] cases with a proved histological diagnosis of hepatitis, seemingly without giant cells.

28 The first of GARCÉS and LEIVA [1954], with a proven diagnosis of neonatal hepatitis with giant cells; the second of LELONG et al. [1961], without diagnostic confirmation of neonatal hepatitis with giant cells.

29 Of HSIA et al. [1958], without diagnostic confirmation of neonatal hepatitis with giant cells.

led some authors [SMETANA *et al.,* 1965, chap. 2] to consider neonatal hepatitis and atresia as a developmental defect, as an expression of a dysgenic etiology ('a congenital disorder of the embryogenesis of undetermined nature and causes' according to the expression of the authors), although of an imprecise type.

However, this pathogenic concept and etiological assumption have had little echo, because: (1) the process is reversible, transitory, at least in a good number of cases, with anatomical and functional recovery of the parenchyma and with the reestablishment of the structure of the liver, both from the canalicular and cellular points of view, and (2) such cells are observed in a great number of diseases of various etiologies, other than hepatitis. At present it is a common belief that such cells are nothing but an acquired dysmorphic-irritative form of the hepatocyte. Recently, they have even been found in another metabolical disease: ornithinemia.

2. Noxa X

In a paper by LAPLANE *et al.* [1964] on familial neonatal hepatitis, they point out that the viral hypothesis seems the most satisfactory because it explains most of the cases reported. However, it also shows uncertain aspects. Nobody up to now, has identified, cultured or innoculated the hepatitis virus: as a result, the authors conclude that perhaps the basis for a viral etiology may be in itself false. Due to this, before endorsing the viral theory, they more prudently refer to a factor X, which is transported in the blood. These authors go on to ask whether the noxious power of this factor would not be due to an immunological phenomenon, a real materno-fetal incompatibility being responsible for neonatal hepatitis, which would be a form of isoimmunization.

3. Isoimmunization

On this subject, PERRIN *et al.* [1966] have published some interesting observations of true isoimmunization, but not of fetal involvement by maternal antibodies. The antibodies found are antitissue antibodies whose specificity, the authors say, is not demonstrated in a sufficient fashion. Due to this, they ask themselves why the liver is more selectively affected: Is it that the liver is more antigenic or, considering that there are differences between tissues in the sense of inducing a transplantation immunity, is the liver more fragile when facing such antibodies?

4. α_1-Antitrypsin, a Trigger Agent or only a Predisposing Cause of Neonatal Hepatitis Frequently Evolving into Cirrhosis?

Cases of neonatal jaundice with frequent evolution into early hepatic cirrhosis [SHARP et al., 1969] as well as neonatal hepatitis with giant cells [JOHNSON and ALPER, 1970] have recently been described where a serum defect in α_1-antitrypsin has been demonstrated.

Is such a defect primarily responsible for a diverse hepatic pathology or is it a predisposing cause to hepatic disorders due to various etiologies (toxic, viral, etc.)? This is a question that in the present state of our knowledge cannot be answered.

C. Discussion of the Objections most Repeatedly Held Up against the Viral-Hepatitis Cause of Neonatal Hepatitis

Although the viral theory of neonatal hepatitis has an increasing number of defenders, there are some objections that have to be answered. Against it is incriminated, in a similar fashion as we have seen for atresia, although with less strength: (1) the fact that a pregnant woman with viral hepatitis gives birth in the majority of cases to a child of healthy aspect, without jaundice, and (2) the fact that neonatal hepatitis can only rarely be directly related with a hepatitic-viral disease of the mother with jaundice during pregnancy or prior to it. Let us see how to answer these objections:

a) The fact that a pregnant woman suffers viral icteric hepatitis[30] need not necessarily mean that she will give birth to a child with hepatitis. It is well known [ZONDECK and BROMBERG, 1947] that *not by far* (the italics are ours) does every epidemic hepatitis of the mother lead to a clinically obvious disease. Recently, SCHMID [1969] has stated: 'A diaplacentarian transmission to the fetus, if it ever does occur, is in all truth exceptional.' Nevertheless, this circumstance does occur, as proved by statistics, both retro and prospectively (pp. 151, 153) [THALHAMMER, 1967]. On the basis of the scarce number of cases in which this contingency occurs, one can be assured that *the incidence of the fetal affection is small.*

This has been clearly confirmed in the prospective review (p. 151) carried out by THALHAMMER [1967] on reports from a good number of authors in which it is stated that, without taking into account the embryos that can be lost during the first

---

30 According to a review of the world literature [SCHMID, 1969], icteric viral hepatitis of the mother is not frequent, as for every 1,500 pregnancies there is only one case of jaundice and 40% of those will be due to viral hepatitis, so that there is approximately 1 case of icteric viral hepatitis/3,750 pregnancies.

Table VI. Fetal risk from maternal hepatitis (epidemic). Compilation of unselected series from Dörfler, Forgacs *et al.*; von Harnack and Martin; Hsia *et al.*, Rath Schubert and Peters Thorling [Thalhammer, 1967]

Result	Trimester		
	I (n=31)	II (n=59)	III (n=92)
Abortions	9	–	–
Stillborns	–	2	3[1]
Prematures	–	3	12
Live-born at term	22	54[2]	77
Of them died at birth	–	1[3]	5[4]
% of dead fetuses	25	5	9

1 Of them 2 before birth.
2 One with n.b. hepatitis.
3 Through n.b. hepatitis.
4 Two of them prematures.

3 months of pregnancy, a *very small number* of fetuses are affected by the mother's viral hepatitis suffered during the course of pregnancy. Of the 173 cases analyzed, 22 corresponded to the first 3 months (having overcome a miscarriage), 59 to the second trimester, and 92 to the last; only two cases corresponding to the second trimester *presented neonatal hepatitis*[31].

This figure certainly does not correspond to the real number, because it refers to fetuses and newborn infants observed during a brief time of their neonatal period – during the days the child remains with the mother in the hospital, a normal postpartum hospitalization of 3–5 days after an uncomplicated delivery. But, if one takes into account, as Alagille and Kremp [1964, chap. 1] point out, that the appearance of jaundice, both for hepatitis and for atresia, occurs during the first week of neonatal life in two thirds of the cases, the result, by means of a simple calculation, will be that *only 2–3% of fetuses whose mothers have suffered epidemic hepatitis during pregnancy will be affected by neonatal hepatitis*. This even depends, we think, mainly but not exclusively (footnote 31) on a hepatitis suffered by the pregnant mother during her second trimester.

From this infrequent affectation of the fetus by a clinically obvious disease of the pregnant mother, a *very low susceptibility* of the fetus and consequently of the newborn can be inferred. This low disposition might

31 These data seem to indicate that the possible pathological contingency for the fetus only exists when the mother suffers hepatitis during the second trimester. As is understandable, a more extensive series is needed to establish this peculiar distribution.

clearly explain the fact that since the disease may be due to viruses A and B, the same mother may produce several affected children, without following a real order of succession [SALAZAR DE SOUZA and SANCHES, 1965, chap. 1].

In the case that occupies us, the situation is probably very similar if not identical to that in chicken pox acquired *in utero* due to maternal disease, which *very rarely* is manifested in the newborn child. This leads us to admit that the *refractoriness of the child would be due to some defense mechanism different to the antibodies,* because the receptivity of the mother is hardly compatible with the transmission of an amount of antibodies sufficient to protect the newborn [NEWMAN, 1965].

The antibodies produced by the mother during the course of the infection, the usual response to every infection, might diminish the risk of disease in the infant. But if there is no sign of disease, not even in an attenuated form, it must be due to the fact that the infant is resistant to it.

Summing up: These data and reasons seem to indicate that if the fetus is affected in such a small proportion of cases, it is because he is *not in a disposition to suffer the disease* in a clinically apparent fashion, with jaundice. It would seem more likely that he is in a situation of being affected in an unapparent, anicteric fashion; a very logical supposition taking into account the known epidemiology of the hepatitis-viral infection and which the recent studies by KRUGMAN *et al.* [1967] experimenting the infection in humans have completely confirmed.

Some authors attribute the infection of the fetus to a placental injury, i.e. no fetal involvement would be possible with an undamaged placenta. Even more, the fetal susceptibility would intrinsically depend on such an eventuality. We believe that probably there would not be fetal involvement without placental lesions. But such a placental lesion would be already a fetal disease, because the trophoblast is an organ of fetal origin formed by the blastodermic layers. For this reason, the placenta considered by many authors as a barrier which could prevent the extension to the fetus, would rather appear to us as a mere way of entry of the infection into the fetus. *For the fetus not to be susceptible there must be an intact placenta.*

The scarce disposition of the fetus to suffer the disease in an apparent way explains, in our opinion, the 6 cases of nonidentical twins reported up to now with only one of the sibs involved in every case. THALHAMMER [1967] interprets this fact in the sense that the disposition to suffer the disease is of 50%; should this be the case, there should have been three instances of involvement of both twins. The fact that there is none clearly indicates that even when the virus was present in all cases (as proved by the affected twin) the other members of the pairs were not susceptible to a clinically obvious disease. Finally, it is logical to explain the circumstance that only one of each of the six pairs of twins was affected considering that the susceptibility to suffer the disease, as we previously said is *only of 2–3%*.

Through this low tendency to the infection, it might be possible to interpret what appears to be the only reported case in identical twins, also with only one of them affected. The small differences that identical twins show in the anatomical functional and pathological fields, might account for a minimal, subtle difference insusceptibility between both twins, so that one became ill and the other did not, or perhaps, that one of them became icterically ill and the other did not.

b) The fact that the majority of cases of neonatal hepatitis occur in babies born to healthy mothers, free from viral hepatitis, does not constitute a solid argument for denying its hepatitis-viral origin. According to THALHAMMER's [1967] retrospective review of 120 cases of hepatitis or cirrhosis[32], in children born to 90 mothers, only 8 of them suffered epidemic hepatitis and only 2 (or perhaps 3) hepatitis due to homologue serum during pregnancy. Of the other 80 mothers giving birth to affected babies (110, because some of them had more than one diseased child) only 5 had suffered hepatitis between 2 and 17 years before. This means that 75 out of the 90 mothers, or 5 out of 6, had never suffered a clinically evident icteric hepatitis.

83% then, in round figures, of mothers who have given birth to one or various children with neonatal hepatitis (or cirrhosis) were not suffering or had never suffered an obvious viral hepatitis. But the virus, in fact, has a greater ubiquity than is generally assumed as proven by two circumstances:

1. Unquestionably, the hepatitis virus not only produces cases clinically manifest with jaundice, but also cases totally asymptomatic, which are apparently more frequent than the former; cases with minimal or no symptoms may be the source of transmission of the virus.

2. It has been convincingly demonstrated that there are persons who for a long time, up to many years, may be carriers of the hepatitis virus due to homologue serum. In pregnant women, according to THALHAMMER [1967], this could be the case in a proportion of 2–3%.

---

32 THALHAMMER's review includes both diseases, neonatal hepatitis and cirrhosis; this second disease is clearly rarer than hepatitis: these are diseases that other authors [BENNET, 1964, chap. 1; THALER, 1964] do not attempt to identify.

These aspects of the peculiar epidemiology and pathology of the hepatitis virus *do not* constitute an obstacle to accepting its causal role in neonatal hepatitis. On the contrary, its incidence, as can be easily perceived, *grossly correlates* with the epidemiological and pathological characteristics of the virus, especially if the scarce fetal susceptibility to it is considered.

We are convinced that this conception would be probably statistically significant; but no statistical analysis has been carried out up to the present moment and we do not know when it will be (although it probably will not take long now, as the hepatitis virus can already be detected with certainty by transmitting it to the marmoset monkey as described by Holmes *et al.* [1966, chap. 5], Köhler and Apodaca [1968, chap. 5], and Apodaca *et al.* [1968, chap. 5]). So far, no reliable figures on the true incidence of the virus in mothers who have given birth to children with hepatitis and in mothers who have given birth to normal children are available.

The same arguments opposed to those who object or completely reject the hepatitic-viral etiology of neonatal hepatitis may be used as the basis to accept that a great majority of cases of atresia can be incriminated to this cause.

1. There are approximately twice as many cases of atresia than of neonatal hepatitis. If between a mother affected by icteric viral hepatitis and an atretic fetus the immunological conditions are the same, i.e. identical correlation between the individual's susceptibility and the agent's virulence, as for a mother affected by such hepatitis and the fetus who will suffer neonatal hepatitis, the number of mothers with hepatitis who would give birth to children with atresia should be *double*. Likewise, the number of calculated cases in Thalhammer's [1967] review should be *double* but in fact there is none.

2. Certainly, it is quite exceptional to find cases of patients with atresia whose mother had suffered icterus-producing hepatitis during pregnancy[33]. In a few cases only, the pregnant mother had suffered it before, i.e. accepting the possibility of the hepatitic-viral etiology of atresia, it would occur that *nearly all the cases of atresia* are born *without an apparent relation* with the hepatitis virus, as are the majority (83%) of those of neonatal hepatitis.

How can one explain this paradox which constitutes the 'black point' to admit the hepatitic-viral etiology of atresia? A possible explanation, in

---

33   In our extensive review of the literature, we found only one case [Tolentino, 1959] and even that was an intrahepatic atresia.

the present state of our knowledge and according to our point of view would be as follows: In clinically evident viral hepatitis of the mother, no cases of atresia occur because the immunological defenses elaborated by her in the course of the disease protect at least *partially* the fetus, avoiding the more extensive necrobiotic injuries and allowing only in the fetus, and later in the newborn, an inflammatory 'atresying' disease of a lesser degree. The cases of atresia occur precisely in pregnant women not apparently ill, or in carriers who produce, or possess, lessened humoral defenses. This point of view of ours is further elaborated from page 171 on.

Conclusions: If one is to admit the hepatitic-viral etiology, according to the clinical data which we possess, the circumstances leading to the development of the fetal disease are as follows: (1) The fetus becomes more seriously affected, *with atresia, practivally in all cases* where the mother is not ill in an apparent way, or is only a carrier. (2) The fetus becomes less seriously affected, *with hepatitis* (a) in the *majority of cases* where the mother is not ill in an apparent fashion or is only a carrier, and (b) in a *minority of cases* where the mother is ill in an apparent fashion.

According to the immunological aspects of the disease currently known both for the epidemic and for the homologue serum hepatitis, if the mother is clinically ill and the child is born *without atresia,* it is because she has developed, in a higher degree than others who carry the disease asymptomatically or are simply carriers, immune phenomena that allow her to successfully overcome the infection. In the usual course of infection there are immunological phenomena, mainly of a cellular nature, as it occurs in viral diseases, but also, to a lesser degree, of a humoral nature.

The antibodies, especially the IgG, may cross the placenta and be influential upon the fetal infection. The γ-globulins, as is already well known, can decrease the severity of the disease and may even prevent the production of jaundice; and this not only in epidemic hepatitis but also in cases due to homologue serum [KRUGMAN and WARD, 1964; MIRICK et al., 1965].

All of this is particularly valid for the B virus, which is the least virulent: less fetal pathogenicity of the B virus as is the case in extrauterine life, according to general opinion.

After discussing the points that to many authors are unquestionable arguments to reject the hepatitic-viral etiology of neonatal hepatitis, particularly in the case of extrahepatic atresia, and before presenting more arguments (pp. 159 ff.) in favor of such an agent as the etiological factor of the triad, let us briefly see how intrahepatic biliary atresia has been considered from an etiological point of view.

III. Intrahepatic Biliary Atresia

The etiology of intrahepatic biliary atresia, an entity even more confusing up to recently than that of its related diseases, extrahepatic atresia and neonatal hepatitis, may be already viewed somewhat more clearly since the acceptance that pathogenically it does not correspond to an ontogenical defect but to a disorganizing process of the ducts, with a variable degree of destruction of the epithelium of the structures that leads to its disappearance unless it is compensated by an adequate regeneration process.

The primary, dysgenic etiology advocated by AHRENS *et al.* [1951, chap. 1] is now amply debated (pp. 126–130). Recently, GHERARDI and MACMAHON [1970], after the observation of two cases in brothers, still admitted the possibility of a genetic basis or dysgenic etiology for intrahepatic atresia and they actually refer to hypoplasia, the term employed by such a great number of authors of the terminal ducts, i.e. of the smallest intrahepatic ones. Nevertheless, the authors accept that they lack the hereditary basis that is so characteristic of other metabolic diseases inherited in a recessive way.

Since BLANC [1962, chap. 5] an increasing number of authors admit the acquired character of intrahepatic biliary atresia. In effect, the two main facts: its frequent association with extrahepatic atresia and its occasional presentation as a particular evolutive process of neonatal hepatitis, lead one to consider that intrahepatic biliary atresia must have a common etiology with the other two entities. Some facts, we believe, would place it in a position closer to extrahepatic atresia: (a) their frequent association, and (b) their uncommon familial presentation, apparently less frequent than in hepatitis, although there is no statistical proof of this point.

In PILLOUD's [1966, chap. 1] review, comprising 42 cases of isolated intrahepatic atresia, there are only two observations with more than one case in a family – that of WILBRANDT and that of HEROLD. Another case that is also included [SWEET, 1932, chap. 2] concerns three observations of extrahepatic atresia in a family with a component of partial intrahepatic atresia in two of them.

The datum of an increased amount of IgM in intrahepatic atresia [FERRANTE and RUBALTELLI, 1971] is also in favor of an acquired infectious process already developed at least in part during intrauterine life.

Special Considerations on Disuse as a Cause of Biliary Atresia

The atrophy of the excretory ducts due to lack of use has been invoked in the production of atresia, especially of the intrahepatic kind. Let us give a detailed account on this subject:

a) For the extrahepatic ducts. AHRENS *et al.* [1951, chap. 1] dismissed it as a mechanism of production of extrahepatic atresia, because there are cases of isolated intrahepatic atresia with normal external ducts. Nevertheless, it is true that when these ducts are not used, as occurs for instance in cases of severe intrahepatic cholestasis, the external ducts can appear clearly 'hypoplasic' or, better, hypothrophic. One of the cholangiographic images of neonatal hepatitis simulating atresia, as pointed out by HAYS *et al.* [1967, chap. 1] is quite demonstrative to this respect.

b) For the intrahepatic ducts. The progressive disappearance of intrahepatic ducts noted in some cases (see p. 88) has been interpreted as due to disuse [COTTON, 1960, chap. 1; KAYE and YAKOVAC, 1962], attributing, however, this disuse to a cholestatic process, i.e. taking it as a secondary etiological cause, subsidiary to another noxa which causes the cholestasis.

We accept that a certain degree of hypotrophy exists or can appear, as 'the function creates the organ' and when an organ does ot function it becomes atrophic. But, to our judgment, in the production determinism of both types of atresia, the basic reason for the decrease, or disappearance of the structures, lies not in the disuse but in a patent morbid action on them; inasmuch as the image which these 'hypoplasic' structures reveal is not that of mere atrophy due to a reduction in size and cellular number, but to an unquestionable process of d-d-n.

IV. Bases of the Viral Etiology of the Triad, with the Hepatitis Virus as the Most Likely Cause

The following points, agreed upon at the European Symposium on Viral Hepatitis (Prage, 1964), must be taken into account for the discussion in this chapter:

1) One should exclusively use the term viral hepatitis, including both epidemic hepatitis and seric hepatitis, *due to the fact that at present there is no sure method* to differentiate between these two diseases, which are clinically (and also pathologically) analogous [DUBIN *et al.*, 1960, chap. 1], although biological and immunobiological features permit to outline the fact that they are two different diseases.

This point of view is still valid according to the ideas of KOHLER *et al.* [1968] based on the studies on the presence and transmission of the virus to the marmoset monkey, the only susceptible animal known so far, and in which there are no biological differences between virus A and B.

2) The propagation mechanisms, exception made of the cases in which seric hepatitis can be confirmed, *are so obscure* that, in general, they are just hypothetical. To those two points we add the following reasonings: There is no specific test for hepatitis, such as for example, the Paul-Bunnell reaction for mononucleosis. A hemaglutination test, a reaction of complement fixation and a cutaneous test have been described but none of them has been proved to be specific. Up to the present moment, a good number of works on the Australia antigen have been published; however, its possible value as a diagnostic tool for viral hepatitis, as well as its etiological role still seem somewhat far from being determined.

Nevertheless, in the present state of our knowledge, the question of the etiology of viral hepatitis and the title to this section does not seem so theoretical any more as a result of the recent experimental studies carried out *in humans* by KRUGMAN *et al.* [1967]. These authors have found common aspects, and at the same time certain differences, between the diseases produced by virus A and B (MS 1 and MS 2, according to their terminology). All this can be briefly outlined as follows:

a) Epidemiology

Serum hepatitis is transmitted by the oral route and through intimate contact, thus denying the concept that up to now considered that it was only rarely transmitted by personal contact. This confirms the idea of previous authors, and especially the work of MIRICK and SHANK [1959], who observed that in an epidemic due to the Sh virus that affected 272 people, another 30 became affected in spite of a lack of parenteral innoculation. This opposes the conception of MACCALLUM [1945] and NEEFE *et al.* [1946] who rejected the oral or intestinal transmission.

b) Clinical and Analytic Data (Humoral Aspects)

Ordinarily the incubation period is longer for seric hepatitis than for epidemic hepatitis. Nevertheless, there are cases of seric hepatitis with a short incubation and, conversely, cases of epidemic hepatitis with a longer period than usual.

In the majority of children studied, aged between 3 and 10 years[34], those who were exposed to contagion or were experimentally inoculated presented anicteric hepatitis. Those who showed jaundice revealed a discreet pigmentation with bilirubin levels between 1 and 3 mg%, beginning to decline in an average period of 5 days. As a result, it is impossible to semiologically differentiate both types of jaundice; this was only possible by means of the following laboratory data: (1) In relation to the increase in serum transaminase activity: the duration of the increase is of only 3–15 days for epidemic hepatitis, while it extends between 35 and 200

34 Very far, then, from infancy and still more from the fetal age, i.e. children in whom the specific susceptibility to the hepatic virus has already increased notably, as observed from the greater morbidity and mortality of the disease.

days with gradual rises and decreases for serum hepatitis. (2) The thymol turbidity reaction is often negative in serum hepatitis (average of 8.5 U), while it is frequently high in epidemic hepatitis (average 15 U).

c) Immunology

Immunity is achieved for the type of infection harbored, but there is no evidence for crossed immunity to occur. That is why the patients with infectious hepatitis do not become immune to serum hepatitis and vice versa. A second bout of hepatitis, according to KRUGMAN *et al.* [1967] takes place in 5.5% of the cases and tends to appear in the first year after the initial episode and even later, up to 7 years, in some cases; this suggests the existence of two immunologically different viruses.

Thanks to the wide range of information provided by the investigations in humans by KRUGMAN *et al.* [1967], the title of this section can be supported by the arguments stated from pages 150 to 155, and furthermore by the following reasons:

1. Admitting an acquired cause, the fact that some familial cases occur in all three entities of the triad would mean that each one of them is not a 'disease of one sole pregnancy', as for example, rubella and toxoplasmosis. And this event would be in agreement with the proven persistence of the hepatitis virus in the human body, especially that of homologue serum, causing no symptoms at all.

2. This happens to be a *causal noxa, preferably attacking the liver*. In effect, neonatal hepatitis is not accompanied by other significant infectious inflammatory manifestations in other organs or systems; these manifestations are not found in atresia either. In the three entities it is possible to find, however, other pathological manifestations of a malformative type. In our opinion, those manifestations would indicate that in such cases, the pathological process began at an early age, during the organogenic period. This, however, would not necessarily imply that in them the hepatopathy began at that stage of the development.

3. That a common etiology should exist at least in some cases of the triad can be seen from what happens in cases of chromosomal aberration (trisomy 18); first, some suffer atresia, neonatal hepatitis or hepatic injuries; second, in others, atresia concomitant with neonatal hepatitis can be demonstrated (p. 139).

4. It is not a chemical toxic agent, because on no occasion a suspicious element of such a nature was found. It has already been indicated that the new and great toxic chemical agent, thalidomide, only produces an aplasia of the gallbladder, but not of the rest of the ducts.

5. A bacterial agent has not been found either. The numerous bacteriological examinations carried out have failed to uncover an agent of this type, either in hepatitis or in atresia.

6. A viral agent therefore must be implicated, similar if not identical with the hepatitis virus. Indeed, there is no other virus so specifically hepatotropic as the hepatitis virus, both of types A and B; in the case of other viruses that can injure the liver, namely the mononucleosis virus, the affinity for this organ is small, and much less prominent than in the case of the hepatitis virus. The hepatitis virus is essentially hepatotropic, whereas the mononucleosis virus is basically lymphoreticulotropic.

The probability of the hepatitic viral etiology of the triad has recently received considerable support after substantial data have been gathered to confirm that another viral disease, maternal rubella, can be responsible for some cases of neonatal hepatitis, as well as of atresia [STRAUS and BERNSTEIN, 1968, chap. 3].

The Australia antigen (HAA)[35] has been studied in neonatal hepatitis and in atresia. The most important facts available today on this subject can be summarized as follows:

a) Routine Investigation of the Antigen in Newborn and Healthy Mothers

The studies by SMITHWICK and GO SUAT CHEN [1970] gave the following results:

1. They did not isolate on any instance the HAA in the cord blood of 2,225 newborns; this is not surprising if the relatively low incidence of atresia and hepatitis are considered.

2. The antigen was investigated in the blood of 271 'normal' mothers, and was found in 6 of them (2.2%); this coincides approximately with the figure of pregnant women to homologue serum virus (p. 153).

3. In 103 cases in which the antigen was simultaneously investigated in mother and child, it was positive in 4 mothers and negative in all the children. Of course, the fact of only demonstrating the HAA in 4 mothers does not eliminate the possibility that this antigen is an etiological agent if one considers that the frequency of diseased children from mothers obviously suffering from hepatitis is very small: 2–3% (p. 151).

35 For the moment it is not possible to identify the hepatitis virus with HAA; perhaps it is included in it, but in any case, in the composition of this antigen, it has not been possible as yet to demonstrate the fundamental element of all living material: nucleic acids.

b) Investigation of the Antigen in Patients Affected by Entities of the Triad

1. With negative result. COSSART [1971] has analyzed 23 cases of neonatal hepatitis and 5 of atresia and the result was negative in all of them. Nevertheless, the following considerations are in order: HAA is found in a large proportion of cases of hepatitis due to homologue serum; with regard to its frequency in epidemic hepatitis, the results are discordant. LONDON *et al.* [1969], GOCKE and KANEY [1969], FARROW *et al.* [1970], and COSSART and VAHRMEN [1970], found nearly the same incidence in both types of hepatitis. On the other hand, according to PRINCE *et al.* [1970], HAA (SH) was found in infections due to virus MS2 and was not found in those due to MS1 or in hepatitis in individuals under 14 years of age, but it is found in a great number of cases of sporadic hepatitis in older people even when they do not have a past history of blood transfusions or other injections. Likewise, SANVALD and SAUERBRUCK [1970] have not found HAA (SH) in 14 cases of epidemic hepatitis in children.

2. With positive result. GILLESPIE *et al.* [1970] found the HAA in a mother and child with neonatal hepatitis. The mother was not clinically ill nor had previously suffered hepatitis or had received any transfusions. TOLENTINO *et al.* [1971] have very recently reported the discovery of the HAA in two cases of partial intrahepatic atresia with extra hepatic agenesia, in which the mothers were also antigen-positive without having presented any symptoms during their pregnancies or offered a past history of hepatitis. In a recent report, FERRANTE and RUBALTELLI [1971] discuss a case of intrahepatic atresia with positive HAA. A curious fact was that the father presented a viral hepatitis 35 days before the child was born.

Latest News on he Antigen Associated to Viral Hepatitis

DEL PRETE *et al.* [1970a], using a new antibody obtained from a multi-transfused patient, have discovered a new antigen[36] which they call 'epidemic hepatitis-associated antigen' (EHAA), also called the 'Milan antigen'.

This antigen was found by DEL PRETE *et al.* [1970b] in 65% of patients from three epidemic outbursts and in 90% of those studied

---

36   Previously, the same author, working together with CONSTANTINO and DOGLIA, had identified in Milan a new antibody which reacts with the conventional Australia antigen, and with the sera from patients suffering from shortly incubated viral hepatitis (epidemic).

during the first 2 weeks of the disease. In these three epidemics, the patients were HAA-negative and this antigen was not found in 2,000 control patients, or in 50 others with various other viral diseases[37].

Following our suggestions, ROBINET-LEVY and LEMAIRE[38] have studied the Australia and Milan antigens in a variety of cases, summarized in table VII.

Summary: Up to now, no definite conclusion can be drawn from the available information on the association of the antigen with viral hepatitis; the hepatitic-viral etiology of neonatal hepatitis and of atresia for the great majority of cases, as we sustain, cannot be confirmed or denied.

7. The specific tropism of the virus for the liver should be manifest at the time the organ shows already some function; this occurs, although slowly, from the third month onwards. The body reacts unspecifically during the embryonic period to other viruses as well, such as the rubella virus, the parotiditis virus (and perhaps others?).

This important question deserves a more detailed discussion:

a) According to the studies of TÖNDURY [1965], carried on by EMMERT [1969], during the first trimester of pregnancy the hepatitis virus will only produce *unspecific* injuries in the fetus: *it does not injure the liver.* Its action, apart from the characteristic 'injuries of the rubella type' (affecting the heart, lens, ear and brain) brings about an illness of a general kind resulting in a miscarriage in a high proportion of cases: in 25%, according to the review carried out by THALHAMMER (table VI). The hepatitis virus would be much more lethal for the embryo than the rubella virus, whose lethality is estimated as 16.4% by MANSON *et al.* [1960]. The higher lethality for the embryo of the hepatitis virus may be readily accepted, considering the higher morbidity of the hepatitis virus in extrauterine life as compared to the rubella virus. On account of its morbous effects on the liver – leading in certain cases of hyperacute hepatitis to hepatic coma – and of its complications, mainly neurolog-

---

37 Nevertheless, later studies cast growing doubt on the antigen specificity, so that at present there are several authors who do not believe in it and discuss its specific nature:

(1) AJDUKIEWICZ, one of the co-workers in DEL PRETE's paper, states that the antigen's specificity is far from clear, as it has been demonstrated in the serum of patients without hepatitis; the antigen may be an indicator of hepatic injury, bearing no relation to any virus, as it is stated in recent works. (2) TAYLOR *et al.* [1972] have apparently defined the antigen as a serum lipoprotein. (3) DEINHARDT [1972] has concluded that EHAA has no relation to viral hepatitis and that the term 'antigen associated with epidemic hepatitis' should be discarded; nor should it be considered as a mere indicator of hepatic involvement, as this lipoprotein can be detected in serum by several methods.

38 From the 'Centre de Transfusion Sanguine Institut d'Hématologie de Montpellier' (France) to whom we are much indebted.

Table VII

	HAA	EHAA
A. Related to extrahepatic atresia		
1. C.G.M. (case 15)	−	
M.M. (mother)	−	−
B. Related to intrahepatic atresia		
1. A.A.A. (not included		
in the series)	−	+ + +
D.A. (mother)	−	−
C. Related to neonatal hepatitis		
1. L.B.V. (case 1)	−	−
M.V. (mother)	−	+
M.B.V. (newborn girl with severe		
physiological jaundice)	−	+ +
2. F.T.P. (case 16)	−	+ + +
M.T. (mother)	−	+
D. Other cases		
1. F.M. (mother of two infants, who		
died with a MacMahon-Thannhauser		
syndrome[1])	−	+
E.M. (father)	−	−
2. J.L.G.A. (congenital hepatic fibrosis)	− [2]	−
A.A. (mother)	+	−

1 Acquired, not congenital type (mentioned on pp. 97 and 196).
2 Already studied 6 months before in another laboratory with a positive result.

ical ones, the hepatitis virus clearly departs from the rubella virus, usually responsible for a clinical picture and types of complications very seldom fatal or severe.

b) To this unspecific *immature* susceptibility of the embryo, basically related to the virulence of the agent, a local predisposing factor would be added in the more *mature* stages of fetal life. The recognition of these two factors does not imply that they play antagonistic roles; quite to the contrary, they are viewed as acting in a sequential manner whenever the initial agression does not lead to the termination of the pregnancy by abortion.

A stage is reached where there is a clear fetal predisposition with a well-defined *organ specificity*. In extrauterine life, once the liver has attained its full maturity and function, the specificity is manifested by the body response to the viral attack, fundamentally consisting in a hepatic injury characterized by a *necrobiotic le-*

sion of the hepatocyte with an accompanying inflammatory reaction, as has been amply demonstrated since the advent of the needle biopsy of the liver.

The evidence offered by these exploratory method has relegated to a very secondary position the previously held theory of the 'mucous plug' as the elementary lesion in the so-called 'hepatitis catarrhalis'.

Therefore, as the fetus matures the susceptibility develops, without reaching the intensity later seen in extrauterine life. *This incomplete response of the fetal liver,* as compared to the pathology commonly seen in extrauterine life is, in our opinion, the essential feature characterizing the action of the hepatitis virus on the biliary tract during the fetal-perinatal period.

Conclusion: The discussion on the objections raised by many authors against the viral hepatitic etiology of neonatal hepatitis and of atresia (pp. 150 ff.), as well as the reasons brought forth on its favor (pp. 159 ff.) seem in our opinion to constitute *very solid ground to accept the hepatitic-viral etiology for a great majority,* if not all, of the *cases of diseases included in the triad.*

V. Systematics of the Embryo and Fetal Pathology

The pathology caused by the hepatitis virus may be either linked to a nonspecific or to a specific susceptibility.

A. Non-specific Susceptibility

The hepatitis virus may produce an *embryopathy* [TÖNDURY, 1965; EMMERT, 1969] with typical or atypical lesions.

1. *Typical,* with the cardinal signs of the 'tetrad', also produced by other viruses, as rubella and parotiditis (and perhaps others?): cataract; injury to the inner ear; cardiac malformations, and cerebral injury (which later is made evident by a mental retardation).

These are frequently accompanied by other less common manifestations of this typical embryopathy, such as: cleft palate; bifid spine; hypospadias, cryptorchidism, etc.

These lesions would possibly be due to a *direct action* of the virus, or more likely to an *indirect action,* resulting in toxic products of carential states for the embryo [THALHAMMER, 1967].

2. *Atypical,* with only some or no malformations of the 'tetrad', and other unusual ones.

To the lesions due to the fetal nonspecific susceptibility, some pathological manifestations induced by a specific susceptibility may be added if the development of the fetus is not interrupted.

B. Specific Susceptibility

This is manifested by a fetopathy, made evident by a hepatopathy which will become patent in the postnatal period.

1. Without obvious clinical signs of disease: *anicteric hepatopathy*.

2. One or more elements of the triad.

From the previous it may be inferred: (a) that necessarily, in a case with triad manifestations with associated malformations, the onset of the lesions must have taken place in the embryonic period, and (b) in the cases without associated malformations, the onset of the disease must be dated in the fetal period.

We rate these statements as postulates, which do not need demonstration. Nevertheless, for the second statement it should be clearly understood that we do not contend that the contagion of the fetus occurred after the embryonic period, already in the frank fetal period. The possibility of a lack of nonspecific susceptibility on the part of the embryo cannot be ruled out, and for this reason it would not have been damaged during the organogenetic period.

Etiological Considerations of the Malformations that can Accompany the Entities of the Triad

As indicated in a previous chapter, the entities of the triad very frequently present accompanying malformations (p. 20). This high correlation between the malformations and the entities of the triad is not random. This fact deserves further consideration so that we can define the exact meaning of this association, which we take as an indication that the entities of the triad often occur in patients with malformations because both are very probably due to the same cause.

1. In *hepatitis* the incidence of association is 13%, so that *a priori* it may be admitted that the hepatitis agent shows a certain preference for the cases with malformations; this is even more obvious if the fact that only 4% of the population suffer ontogenical defects is taken into account. On the other hand, it may be argued that 87% of the cases of hepatitis appear in the remaining 96% of the population, free from congenital malformations. From this data one may validly infer that the cases of hepatitis recognize only one etiology (acquired) whereas the cases with

the association of malformations and hepatitis should be attributed to two separate noxious agents: one responsible for the embryological disorder and the other causing the inflammatory process.

One can conclude that hepatitis takes place in malformed patients by other causes, or that the malformations are a result of the same causal agent of hepatitis. Arguments in favor of the latter possibility are:

a) It has been demonstrated that the cause held responsible for the inflammation, the hepatitis virus, *can induce it*. This is supported by THALHAMMER's compilation of various precious retrospective reports (p. 153), and the same author's compilation of a good number of reports studied prospectively (p. 151).

b) It has also been demonstrated that this virus is teratogenic [TÖNDU-RY, 1965; EMMERT, 1969]. Therefore, it would seem as more logical to assume that the same agent can act in the production of both disorders; perhaps some cases do not fit into this explanation, but it does seem the most logical interpretation for the majority of cases. The true congenital malformations, accidental deformities excepted, imply an embryological disorder; their association to inflammatory manifestations would be the result of a noxious agent acting at two different moments of intrauterine life.

2. The same considerations we have made for hepatitis are valid for *atresia* of both extrahepatic and intrahepatic types, and more so for the latter where there is a larger number of associated malformations. It should be pointed out, however, that only in very rare instances has it been possible to correlate atresia with a hepatoviral disease of the mother as an antecedent to the disease. We found only a report of one case in which the mother, having suffered hepatitis during pregnancy, gave birth to a child with intrahepatic atresia [TOLENTINO, 1959]. Nevertheless, we think that attention is due to the recent demonstration by TOLENTINO *et al.* [1971] of HAA in two cases of partial intrahepatic atresia with extra agenesia both in the babies and in their mothers, who had not shown any symptoms during pregnancy and did not have a past history of hepatitis. FERRANTE and RUBALTELLI [1971] have made a similar observation.

VI. Frequency and Prognosis of the Infection of the Embryo and the Fetus by the Hepatitis Virus

The pathological involvement of the embryo or the fetus during intrauterine life must be analyzed in two different situations: with icteric maternal hepatitis in the course of pregnancy, or with anicteric hepatitis or in a carrier state.

A. With Icteric Hepatitis During Pregnancy
1. Epidemic Hepatitis Virus
Two separate sets of effects of this agent must be considered, in relation to a nonspecific or a specific embryonic or fetal susceptibility:

a) Corresponding to the nonspecific susceptibility. They constitute the cases of great severity in which the affected embryos show little or no resistance, according to data drawn from the review by THALHAMMER [1967], from reports of a good number of authors (quoted in table VI), and that of DÖRFLER [1957].

When the mother has suffered a clinically obvious epidemic hepatitis during the first trimester of pregnancy, the lethal action of the virus is as high as 25%. The remaining 75% seem to escape infection, with a very few number of cases that show congenital malformations, without signs of hepatopathy, attributable to the virus of epidemic hepatitis that caused the disease of the mother during the first 3 months of pregnancy [DÖRFLER, 1957]. One half of these cases reveal some signs of typical viral embryopathy accompanied by other unusual malformations, and the other half presents malformations which do not belong to the 'tetrad'.

75% of the embryos reach the term of pregnancy without any obvious pathology; this conclusion has been drawn from a statistic of 22 out of 31 cases at term with 9 miscarriages.

This ratio cannot be considered as an exact figure although it certainly must be very approximate, as the number of embryos that resist the viral attack due to a lack of nonspecific susceptibility and which later will be at risk due to a possible specific susceptibility is very small: only 22 cases. This figure is also too exiguous to allow the conclusion that once the first trimester is over, the fetus *always* remains undamaged, because according to the same review by THALHAMMER [1967], the incidence in the second trimester is very low too, with only 2 cases (or 3 according to the correction of the figures indicated on p. 151) being involved.

b) Corresponding to a specific susceptibility. These are less frequent, and seldom lethal.

Due to epidemic hepatitis of the mother acquired in the second trimester: (a) The perinatal mortality is not influenced by the maternal process; (b) it is not a cause of prematurity, and (c) out of the 59 cases collected by THALHAMMER [1967], only two suffered hepatitis, or with the corrected figure, 3; i.e. 5.5%.

Due to epidemic hepatitis of the mother acquired during the third trimester: (a) This does not seem to influence the antenatal mortality, but it may somewhat affect the natal mortality; (b) marked increase of prematurity, and (c) in the 92 collected cases neither a case of neonatal hepatitis nor of cirrhosis was found. Accepting that due to the short neonatal period of observation some cases could be missed, it can be assumed that the risk of suffering a clinically obvious hepatopathy due to specific susceptibility motivated by the icteric epidemic hepatitis of the mother during the third trimester can be approximately of 1–2%.

c) Due to a mixed susceptibility. This would be in cases of hepatitis or atresia with associated malformations. Compared to the cases that showed an exclusive specific susceptibility, the number of cases of hepatitis or atresia with accompanying malformations constitutes, as previously indicated (pp. 20 ff.), a small proportion. The figures given by ALAGILLE and KREMP [1964, chap. 1] and ALAGILLE et al. [1969, chap. 1], who are the only ones who have evaluated them in the three entities, are the following: 13% in hepatitis; 23% in extrahepatic atresia, and a greater figure for intrahepatic atresia, in which, according to these authors, 28% presented cardiac malformations.

The fact of having escaped miscarriage indicates quite clearly that the developmental defects in such cases have been of little or no importance for the survival of the embryo or the fetus.

2. Homologue Serum Hepatitis Virus

We do not possess extensive and precise data about the frequency and severity of the risks to the embryo or the fetus if the pregnant woman suffers from serum hepatitis. It would appear, though, that such a virus could be responsible for cases of hepatitis, and/or cirrhosis of the newborn, according to the retrospective review by THALHAMMER [1967]. According to reports collected up to 1944, the course of pregnancy in cases of hepatitis or cirrhosis of the newborn is as follows:

Epidemic hepatitis	Serum hepatitis	No hepatitis
8	2 (or +1?)	110

Also according to data of ELLEGAST et al. [1954a, b], the patent serum hepatitis during pregnancy can behave essentially in the same way as epidemic hepatitis.

These authors found 57 such pregnant women who suffered hepatitis due to homologous serum; out of these there were 15 premature deliveries with 4 of these babies dying shortly afterwards and 2 stillbirths.

Another 4 women gave birth in the prodromic state of the disease; they gave birth to 1 stillborn and to 3 prematures, in 3 cases 2 weeks before the onset of jaundice, and in 1 case just 1 week before its onset. This amounts to a total fetal loss of 15%. Nevertheless, as autopsies were not carried out, the pathology of these fetuses remains unknown.

B. With Anicteric Hepatitis or a Carrier State of the Mother

In the present state of our knowledge, the future pathology of the fetus when the pregnant woman is affected by anicteric hepatitis due to one or another virus or being a carrier is not known. This is due to the fact that such pathological or parapathological states can only be diagnosed virologically, a method that has not been applied as yet. It can be assumed, however, that the disease of fetus depends essentially on its susceptibility.

1. Corresponding to a nonspecific susceptibility. The number of cases of miscarriage or malformation will not be as low as one could suppose because:

a) It is universally admitted that the number of cases of viremia without clinical evidence is much higher than the number of cases with patent symptomatology (with jaundice) and that a carrier state for this virus is possible although it does not seem to be frequent.

b) It is also commonly accepted that a viremia mostly due to the B virus does occur in pregnant women, with an incidence given by THALHAMMER [1967] as 2–3%; this would fall within the figures admitted for the general population quoted between 0.5 and 6%.

2. Corresponding to a specific susceptibility. Admitting the etiological role of the hepatitis virus in the triad and taking into account the general biological law that a disease does not take place unless there is an individual disposition, as statistically proven, the number of cases of atresia and neonatal hepatitis related only to viremia due to the A and B viruses should be higher than the number of cases presenting in pregnant women with icteric hepatitis. This leads one to consider the following section.

VII. Discussion of the Hypothesis Relating the Type of Virus with the Entities of the Triad – The A Virus with Atresia (Extrahepatic) and the B Virus with Hepatitis

At this point, it seems pertinent to ask: Could one assign to each type of hepatitis virus a predominant or exclusive role in the causality of the entities of the triad: one virus for hepatitis and another for atresia? Before entering into the consideration of such an important point (p. 177), let us see some other aspects which we deem of the utmost interest.

A. Onset and Development of the Triad During Intrauterine Life

The facts discussed in previous chapters lead us to admit that the fetopathy which will eventually lead to a hepatopathy manifested by one or more of the entities of the triad begins, in a small proportion of cases (those that will show associated malformations in other organs), during the embryonic period, i.e. as an embryopathy. The majority of cases start well into the fetal period; usually, although not exclusively, in the second trimester.

This fetopathy will evolve in the course of some months, up to a maximum of six (this would be the whole fetal life), for those who are born at term presenting associated developmental defects.

Usually, this fetopathy will not hinder the formation of a normal meconium which should contain enough bilirubin or biliverdin (mainly the former) to give it a black-green color. As is well known, this pigment is elaborated mostly from the seventh month onwards, during the eighth, and above all during the ninth month, as was already stated by YLPPÖ [1913, chap. 5].

This hepatopathy follows a protracted course, and does not reach a *period of state or cholestatic state* until after the meconium has already acquired a normal color in the majority of cases. Later on, the hepatopathy will be manifested by its capital sign, jaundice, within the first week of postnatal life in two thirds of the cases.

The functional damage caused by such a hepatopathy appears to be of little importance, judging by the fact of the normally colored meconium, which we admit is pigmented exclusively or predominantly by the bile secretion (see physiology of the pigmentation of the meconium, pp. 114 ff.). This could evidence that the liver has been secreting and the ducts have remained patent until the late stages of pregnancy, or even in some cases up to the moment of birth. Only in the cases with an abnormally colored meconium, i.e. without is characteristic dark green hue, as has been observed in a few cases of both atresia and hepatitis, will it be reasonable to admit that the hepatopathy was already cholestatic from an earlier period of the fetal life, certainly before the beginning of the eighth month.

How can we explain, then, such a slow evolution of the disease during pregnancy and its 'burst' with a deep jaundice, during the first days or weeks of life?

It is difficult to give a completely satisfactory explanation of it, although the following reasonings seem quite logical:

a) The maternal immunobiological conditions, specifically the humoral defensive mechanisms, cannot be unrelated to the course of this hepatopathy. In fact, the γ-globulin, especially its G fraction, possesses a well-demonstrated antihepatic-viral action.

But, as KRUGMAN et al. [1967] have confirmed, the γ-globulin does *not* prevent hepatitis, but only lessens its severity, without significantly shortening its course, reducing the number of *icteric* hepatitis in adults and schoolchildren in 85%. The γ-globulin, as documented by PAKTORIS [1966] in more than 600,000 schoolchildren, reduces the number of cases of hepatitis, both icteric and anicteric, although the proportion for these two types increases in favor of the latter.

The presence of circulating antibodies reduces or controls the infection which can be reactivated when their levels decrease or their production ceases.

This occurs, for example in patients who possess antibodies against the cytomegalovirus and receive an allograft. With the immunosuppressive treatment to prevent rejection, a high incidence of complications by this virus occurs [CRAIGHEAD et al., 1967; MUNK and RUNNEBAUM, 1970]. But as in every viral disease, the fight against the agent and the establishment of immunity depend not only of the humors, but especially on the cells themselves; the antibodies bound to the globulins are insufficient on their own to control the infection.

A logical partial protection can be attributed to the *mother's G immunoglobulin with its corresponding antibodies,* on account of the fact that the mother is suffering an infection, patent or not evident, or she has previously suffered it and maybe she is still a carrier, especially in the case of the type B virus, *transmitting it to the fetus* through the placenta.

The placentary transmission to children of infectious hepatitis during pregnancy is frankly unusual, as the children are probably protected by maternal γ-globulins [SHERLOCK, 1963, chap. 1]. Thus, this partial protection substantially decreases the severity of the process while the fetus remains *in utero*. Immediately after delivery, the fetus will be fighting on its own without the contribution of the maternal immunoglobulin. On the other hand, the IgG levels in the infant decrease rapid and progressively [23 days of half-life – MIETENS, 1971]; and if one takes into account that the production of G globulin does not begin until the second month after birth and that it is produced in a moderately ascensional rhythm (very much below the M γ-globulin which also contributes with an anti-infectious but less efficient action), it will be understood why the course of the hepatitic-viral infection is usually long. The inability of the infant to produce IgG is indicated by STOWENS [1966, chap. 2] as one of the causes of neonatal hepatitis (with giant cell transformation) that usually folows a long course.

Furthermore, we think that the special immunological situation of each individual case would be the commanding factor in the determinism of each of the entities of the triad. It would seem that an eventually favorable evolution of the fetal lesions should be described to the presence of viral antibodies bound to the IgG produced by the pregnant woman who is fighting, usually with success, against the infection, as these antibodies can usually cross the placenta, and perhaps also arise from the antiviral antibodies elaborated by the fetus itself and involved in the IgM fraction. This has also been demonstrated in the case of the rubella virus, another agent capable of producing hepatitis and atresia.

Logically, the presence of the antibodies of the IgG and IgM fractions must bring forth an attenuation of the infection, and a decrease of the atresia-inducing action of the pathological noxa.

On the other hand, when there is an antibody deficiency – be it in pregnant women who do not suffer the disease in an apparent form, or in women carriers with smaller production of antibodies or, finally in women who did suffer previously the infection, but in whom circulating antibodies have already disappeared – the contribution of defensive elements does not take place or is inadequate so that the susceptible fetus may suffer more severe inuries.

b) The postnatal 'burst' of the disease will likewise be significantly influenced by the demand of a larger amount of bile secretion needed for the digestive work, absent up to then. This increase in bile secretion was already quantified by YLPPÖ [1913, chap. 2] many years ago, precising that the production of bile pigment in the first 5 days of postnatal life equals that in the last 2 months of intrauterine life.

The physiological disorder that explains the production of a retentive icteric syndrome will have to be fundamentally attached to the larger amount of bilirubin, mostly of the direct type, elaborated by the liver, whose excretion will be hindered in the diseased viscus.

B. Special Considerations on why the Newborn is not Jaundiced

It is a known fact that a newborn does not become jaundiced with blood bilirubin levels of 1.5–2 mg% as it would happen with an older child or with an adult. A higher level, from 8 to 9 mg%, is required to produce a latent staining of the tissues. This fact, pointed out by several authors, still awaits a satisfactory explanation [WITH, 1968, chap. 1].

Why does not a child suffering hepatitis or atresia present at birth a higher blood bilirubin level producing a cutaneous and conjunctival pigmentation? We think it can be explained as follows:

a) When the severity of the process *in utero* ought to cause a staining of the tissues, *this does not become evident* due to the following reasons:

1. The direct bilirubin elaborated by the hepatic cell flows back into the bloodstream; as it cannot be eliminated via the diseased liver, *it is excreted through the placenta.* The indirect bilirubin, which can increase later on due to a more or less severe involvement of the conjugation system, is easily excreted by the placental route as well.

But is it possible for the placenta to eliminate *direct* bilirubin? It has been said that only a minimal amount may pass through it [SHENKER *et al.*, 1964, chap. 5, in studies in guinea pigs; LESTER *et al.*, 1963, chap. 5, in studies in monkeys]; however, if a certain amount does pass, it will have to be accepted that this 'minimal amount' does not equal nil.

2. If it is categorically denied that the placenta allows the passage of fetal direct bilirubin to the mother, *its elimination through urine* will have to be admitted. This actually occurs in extrauterine life before the blood bilirubin reaches a high level and before the skin pigmentation becomes manifest, as is well known.

In such a situation, the direct bilirubin drained into the ammiotic fluid will be ingested by the fetus. This will stain the meconium even further *unless it is absorbed by the intestine.* Clinical studies in adults and experimental studies on animals [LESTER *et al.*, 1963, chap. 5; SCHMID, 1969] have proved that the intestine can absorb direct bilirubin, although it must be previously deconjugated. This requires the presence in the digestive tract of an active enzyme system to direct such a process. The presence of a large amount of β-glucuronidase in the meconium [BRODER-SEN and HERMANN, 1962], which decreases rapidly during the first days of life, would prove the existence of such a system.

3. Perhaps both the placental and the urinary routes, contributing to the elimination of direct bilirubin, account for the absence of jaundice in the newborn.

b) In fact, the process *in utero does not reach the severity required to cause pigmentation* of the tissues. We believe this to be the most common occurrence on account of the following reasons:

1. Considering that cholestasis means elaboration of bile whose excretion is interfered with by the pathological process, a cholestasis severe enough to cause pigmentation of tissues does not seem very likely, as the liver function appears to be very limited in the late stages of intrauterine life.

2. Another significant reason is, in our opinion, that the pathological process, hepatitis or atresia, do not produce a complete cholestasis, because *the process has not reached its peak,* and the altered biliary excre-

Table VIII. Possible pathological manifestations due to the hepatitis virus in the various periods of pregnancy

---

A. Patent maternal viremia (with jaundice)

  1. In the first trimester
     a) Abortions: 25% (observed in cases of epidemic hepatitis) attributed to an unspecific disposition
     b) The pregnancies not interrupted may reach term with a newborn who may present some malformations; there is, in this group, *a low incidence* of cases presenting one of the entities of the triad attributed to a specific disposition

  2. In the second and third trimesters
     a) No abortions: There is an increased rate of prematurity and perinatal mortality
     b) *The fetuses can also be specifically affected by* the entities of the triad, but *in a low proportion,* although it is *higher for the second trimester*[1]. In maternal epidemic hepatitis suffered in the second trimester of pregnancy, there is an incidence of 5.5% of neonatal hepatitis

B. Viremia not patent (without jaundice[2])

  1. First trimester
     a) The proportion of abortions is not known as the incidence of viremia is also unknown, *although it is probably high, similar to that of apparent viremia, because the disease of the embryo depends essentially on its unspecific disposition*
     b) *Those cases escaping abortion are in the situation of A.1b)*

  2. For the second and third trimesters *same as for A.2. a) and b)*

---

1 It is admitted that the onset of the fetal disease may correspond to the third trimester, as this is known to occur, for example, with polio [THALHAMMER, 1967].
2 Symptomless anicteric hepatitis with some signs occasionally present: hepatomegaly, a raise in serum transaminase levels, etc., or a maternal 'carrier state'. NB: The *italics* are ours.

---

tion *has not impeded,* in the majority of cases, the elaboration of a normal meconium.

There are therefore several mechanisms to explain the lack of manifest jaundice at birth in a fetus affected by triad. The jaundice becomes obvious shortly after birth because: (a) the placentary route of excretion no longer exists; (b) the bile retention is greater because the liver elaborates more bile, and (c) the pathological process has increased in severity, becoming more cholestatic. As a corollary, it can be accepted that when

Table IX. Comparison of antenatal risks in rubella and hepatitis

---

A. Risks to the embryo

    1. Rubella: Morbidity 25–30%
       Half of these terminate in abortion[1]. The other half is born with malforma-
       tions and other specific manifestations: exanthema, purpura, etc., if the
       noxious action of the virus continues during the fetal period

    2. Hepatitis (referred to epidemic hepatitis): Morbidity 25%
       The vast majority terminate in abortion. *A very small proportion escape, some*
       of them presenting malformations, and can later become ill in a specific manner
       with a hepatic injury (triad)

B. Risks to the fetus

    1. Rubella: Slight risk apparently due to a greater virulence of the virus. The
       'syndrome of neonatal rubella' with typical lesions and some unusual ones
       (hepatitis) has been reported in certain American areas; even malformations
       may appear when the onset of the disease dates back to the embryonic period.
       Its capacity for producing atresia seems to be demonstrated

    2. Hepatitis: Slight risk. It may possibly cause hepatitis (or cirrhosis)
       and rarely, atresia

---

1 This high incidence of abortions is even higher in the case of polio [47%, according
to THALHAMMER 1967]. According to TÖNDURY [1965], the majority of these abortions
are due to embryopathies. NB.: The figures are from THALHAMMER [1967], in his
extensive review. The *italics* are ours.

---

in a case of atresia, the jaundice takes more than a week to become manifest and the feces become acholic beyond 10 days after birth, *atresia has*
started in the postnatal period.

This is how DANKS [1969, chap. 1] judges three of this observations in which
he demonstrated the presence of colored feces between the tenth day and the seventh week after birth; this is what we think occurred in our cases numbers 3, 5, 10,
12, and 15. These observations constitute examples of the apparently postnatal development of atresia pointed out years ago by some authors [KAYE *et al.*, 1957,
chap. 5; HOLDER, 1964, chap. 5].

Summary: The fact that a newborn affected by hepatitis or atresia
does not show jaundice at birth results from several factors, although at
present it is not possible to incriminate any single one of them as the main
or sole responsible. Nevertheless, we believe it can be asserted with little
possibility of error that for the cases that become jaundiced after the first

week of life, and especially those that present jaundice in two consecutive periods, the peak of the pathological process was not reached until the time of presentation of cholestasis, as made evident by the obvious jaundice: this would happen only in full extrauterine life.

C. Chronopathology of Hepatitis Virus Compared with that of Rubella

The chronopathology of the hepatitis virus (table VIII) will be better understood if compared with that of the rubella virus (table IX).

D. Moment of Action of the Supposed Etiological Agents – The A and B Hepatitis Viruses

a) The *overall incidence* of congenital malformations without explainable cause is of 4%, according to LUNDSTRÖM [1962, chap. 1][39].

b) The *frequency of association malformations* in each of the entities of the triad [figures provided by ALAGILLE and KREMP, 1964, chap. 1, and ALAGILLE et al., 1969, chap. 1, the only authors who have given them for the three entities]: in extrahepatic atresia, 23%; in neonatal hepatitis, 13%; and in intrahepatic atresia, the cardiac malformations alone constitute 28%. From this data the following statements can be drawn:

1. In *extrahepatic atresia*, the fact that in 23% of the cases malformations are present can be interpreted as: (a) That in 19%, or perhaps up to 23% of the cases, if this 4% of unexplained malformations could be attributed to the same agent, the disease will have affected the fetus during the first trimester of pregnancy (or during the first 4 months according to

39   This figure corresponds to *all* the malformations observed in live births who have been followed for a period of 1–3 years; the same figure has been given by BUZARD and CONKLIN [1964]. It represents the average of values given by other authors; in effect, as TÖNDURY [1965] indicates, the percentage of macroscopic malformations that can be estimated at the end of pregnancy or can be demonstrated by anatomical examination including stillborns and children who die after delivery is from 1 to 1.5%. For all children born after 28 weeks of pregnancy and kept under observation during a period of 1 year after delivery, the number of malformations increases to 4 or 5%. NEEL [1958] examined 16,144 infants of 9 months of age and found important malformations in 3.12%, whereas MCINTOSH et al. [1954] in a group of 5,739 children, found 7.5%. According to LAMY and FRÉZAL [1960] the value given by NEEL [1958] is too low, and the one given by MCINTOSH et al. [1954] seems to be excessively high. If we include in the total figures, the malformations which will later manifest themselves in youth or adulthood, according to LAMY and FRÉZAL [1960] the total will amount to 5–6%. This figure does not include the many fetuses that died inside the uterus due to malformations.

the concept of embryonic period of THALHAMMER). (b) That in the remaining 77% (or perhaps 81% if the indicated malformations are not attributed to the hepatitis virus), the disease must have started after the first trimester.

2. In *neonatal hepatitis,* the fact that 13% of the cases present malformations means that: (a) In 9% of the cases (or 13%, if the 4% of the malformations which are considered of an unknown etiology can be attributed to the hepatitis virus), the initiation of the process affecting the fetus takes place during the first trimester. (b) in 87% of the cases (or 91%) the disease will have begun beyond the first trimester of pregnancy.

3. In *intrahepatic atresia.* The lack of exact figures prevents us from predicting with precision the moment of onset of the disease, but it appears that the number of cases beginning in the organogenetic period is higher than in extrahepatic atresia if the figures of malformations correspond to true cardiac malformations and not to involutive defects (especially patent ductus).

E. Data in Favor of a Preferential Etiology for Hepatitis and Atresia
Hepatitis is mainly caused by the B virus and atresia is mostly due to the A virus.

According to PILLOUD's [1966, chap. 1] hypothesis, atresia would be the expression of a more precocious fetal injury. We take issue with this point of view because if we accept it, many more cases of atresia with discolored meconium, if not all of them, would be observed, and this is in conflict with the data of ALAGILLE and KREMP [1964, chap. 1].

Nonetheless, there are some elements in atresia which reveal a greater morbus intensity of the agent; among them: (1) the lesion itself, the d-d-n process, is more severe; (2) there are more associated malformations revealing a higher nonspecific susceptibility that relatively or absolutely corresponds to a greater morbidity of the causal noxa.

In table X, we expose an etiological hypothesis partly modifying the JONES *et al.* [1968, chap. 1] concepts.

a) This etiological hypothesis is essentially based on the following arguments: (1) the majority of cases, even though presenting the pathological findings of the inflammatory and atresia-inducing disease, can be classified in a specific entity; (2) it is generally admitted that the B viremia lasts much longer than the A viremia; (3) the frequent familial character of hepatitis, rarely observed in atresia, especially of the extrahepatic type, and (4) the more serious damage caused by the A virus.

Table X. Etiological hypothesis, partly following the concepts of Jones et al. [1968, chap. 1]

Entity	Producing agent	Mother's viremia conditions	Familial presentation	Parents' consanguinity	Mal-for-ma-tions
Extrahepatic biliary atresia	A virus	obvious in exceptional cases (icteric hepatitis)? In the vast majority, not obvious	very unusual because the viremia is of short duration	no	in 23%
Neonatal hepatitis	B virus	in the majority, not obvious	a good number of cases, because the viremia lasts longer	yes[1]	in 13%
Intrahepatic biliary atresia	A and B viruses; greater probability for the A virus?	?	in some cases	?	more than 28%[2]

1 The figures available up to date have not been statistically evaluated (p. 19).
2 Unclassified heart defects, corresponding, it seems, to the sum of true developmental malformations and simple evolutionary defects (e.g. ductus botali).

b) Other data may be considered against the general acceptance of this etiological hypothesis which would be valid only for most, but not for all, cases. The most important objections to the exclusive single etiology of these entities are:

1 The fact that the familial presentation of extrahepatic atresia also occurs indicates that: (a) if the A virus causes a viremia of a short duration, the B virus should also be responsible for the production of atresia, and (b) if we admit that the A viremia can also be longlasting, as Aterman [1963, chap. 3] has indicated, this virus can then be considered as the cause of hepatitis.

Certainly the possibility, and even the probability, that each hepatitic virus can produce two very similar pathoclinical entities is in agreement with the studies of Dubin et al. [1960, chap. 1], according to which both the A and B viruses can be responsible, in the adult, of one or the oher type of hepatitis: the usual (ordinary) and the cholestatic types. This is not in disagreement with the investigations of KRUGMAN *et al.* [1967], who have underlined how these viruses offer clear differential features only from the immunological point of view.

2 There are cases difficult to asign to a specific hepatitis virus. This occurs in cases of different entities presenting in the same family e.g. one of hepatitis and another of extrahepatic atresia [ALAGILLE *et al.*, 1969, chap. 1; GUBERN-SALISACHS, 1968, chap. 5]. These cases, however, can be explained without exceeding the indicated etiological presumption. It seems to be well established that there is no cross-immunization between these two viruses.

As a confirmation of this statement we can cite one of our cases of neonatal hepatitis which had been surgically explored, cured without sequelae and at the age of 4 years suffered an epidemic hepatitis. This concept would imply that the source of infection would have included through not necessarily at the same time, the two viruses. Otherwise, we will have to accept that one and the same virus can cause both entities.

As for the extremely exceptional familial cases, in which the three entities are present independently – as in a case reported by ALAGILLE *et al.* [1969, chap. 1] – which etiology can be assigned to them? Really, there will be few who in this circumstance will dare give another explanation than the exclusive role of the individual as a determining element of each of the entities.

3 Which cause do we ascribe to the mixed cases with two coincidental entities, usually hepatitis and extrahepatic atresia [for example, the case of SCOTT *et al.*, 1954, chap. 2]? Will one have to accept that both viruses act simultaneously? Can the individual show two susceptibilities at the same time? Our opinion is that there is little doubt that the responsible agent will be only one of the viruses, more likely the A virus; and that the cases with a mixed pathoclinical picture only constitute an expanded result (complete in the case where the three entities are found together) of the inflammatory and atresia-inducing disease.

Finally, to which etiology can the *intrahepatic biliary atresia* be incriminated? Can a predominant producing agent be assigned to it?

It is true that intrahepatic atresia, which in many aspects (clinical, biological, pathological, etc.) occupies an intermediate situation among its related diseases, should be equally considered at an intermediate level from an etiological point of view, as far as it seems in the present state of our knowledge.

1. It cannot be considered as a clear, frank atresia like the extrahepatic type, because should this be the case, there would be less familial cases, whereas what really occurs is that there are relatively more.

2. It cannot be considered as a mere hepatitis either, because in such a case the number of familial cases should be greater.

This point, nevertheless, remains undecided for the moment, due to the relatively scarce number of observations reported. For such reasons, and in a provisional manner, the etiological assignation is temporarily that shown in table IX.

Conclusion: Although there are still certain doubts about the etiology of the triad, especially in the case of each of the entities, the fact that the same hepatitis virus can be incriminated as etiological agent for the various entities, and especially the fact that an individual disposition would constitute the prime factor in determining their clinical manifestations, are arguments of undeniable value in the concept of the inflammatory and atresia-inducing disease and very particularly of its pathogeny.

References

AJDUKIEWICZ, A. B.; FOX, R. A.; DUDLEY, F. J.; DONIACH, D., and SHERLOCK, S.: Immunological studies in an epidemic of infective short-incubation hepatitis. Lancet i: 803 (1972).

ALPERT, L. I.; STRAUSS, L., and HIRSHORN, K.: Neonatal hepatitis and biliary atresia associated with trisomy 17–18 syndrome. New Engl. J. Med. 280: 16 (1969).

BING, C.: Virchows Arch. path. Anat. Physiol. 35: 360 (1866); cit. THOMPSON (Edinb. med. J. 37: 523, 604, 724, 1112 (1891–92) and SWEET.

BLATTNER, R. J.: Coxsackie virus infection. J. Pediat. 68: 315 (1966).

BODIAN, M. et NEWNS, G. H.: Hépatitie néo-natale. Archs fr. Pédiat. 10: 169 (1953).

BUTLER, L.; SNODGRASS, G. A. T.; FRANCE, N. E.; SINCLAIR, L., and ARSELL, E.: (16–18) Trisomy syndrome. Analysis of 13 cases. Archs Dis. Childh. 40: 600 (1965).

BUZARD, F. and CONKLIN, A.: Tuberculostatics, sulfonamides and antibiotics. Am. J. Physiol. 206: 189 (1964).

CLAIREAUX, A. E.: Neonatal hyperbilirubinaemia. Br. med. J. i: 1528 (1960).

COLE, A. R.; PURDUE, B. S.; DANKS, D. M., and CAMPBELL, P. E.: Hepatitis virus in neonatal liver disease. Lancet i: 1138 (1965).

COSSART, Y. E.: Personal commun. in the discussion to her lecture on Australian antigen, Barcelona 1971.

COSSART, Y. E. and VAHRMAN, J.: Studies of Australia-SH antigen in sporadic viral hepatitis in London. Br. med. J. i: 403 (1970).

CRAIGHEAD, J. E.; HANSHAW, J. B., and CARPENTER, C. B.: Cytomegalovirus infection after renal allotransplantation. J. Am. med. Ass. 201: 725 (1967).

DEINHARDT, F. W.: An epidemic of infective short-incubation hepatitis. Lancet *i:* 1118 (1972).

DÖRFLER, R.: Zur Frage der kindlichen Missbildungen infolge Erkrankungen der Mutter an Hepatitis Epidemica während der Schwangerschaft. Münch. med. Wschr. *99:* 1664 (1957).

EDWARDS, J. H.; HARNDEN, D. G.; CAMERON, A. H.; GROSSE, V. M., and WOLF, O. H.: A new trisomic syndrome. Lancet *i:* 787 (1960).

ELLEGAST, H.: GRUMPESGERGER, G. und WEWALKER, F.: Hepatitis in der Gravidität und Frühgeburt. Wien. klin. Wschr. *66:* 30 (1954a).

ELLEGAST, H.; GRUMPESGERGER, G. und WEWALKER, F.: Einfluss einer Hepatitis in der Schwangerschaft auf das Kind. Wien. klin. Wschr. *66:* 507 (1954b).

EMMERT, A.: Virushepatitis und Keimschädigung. Über histologische Veränderungen an Keimlingen, deren Mütter während der Schwangerschaft an Virus hepatitis erkrankten. Z. Kinderheilk. *105* (1969).

FARROW, L. J.; HOLBROW, E. H.; JOHNSON, G. D.; LAMB, S. G.; STEWART, T. S.; TAYLOR, P. E., and ZUCKERMAN, A.: Auto-antibodies and the hepatitis-associated antigen in acute infective-hepatitis. Br. med. J. *ii:* 693 (1970).

FERRANTE, L. and RUBALTELLI, F. F.: Intrahepatic biliary atresia associated with the presence of Australia antigen. Pädiat. Pädol. *6:* 225 (1971).

FRIESEL, E. and LUNDQUIST, C. W.: Jättecellshepatit hos spädbarn. Nord. Med. *54:* 1459 (1955); cit. ATERMAN (chap. 3).

GAL, G.: Beiträge zur Pathologie der Hepatitis im Säuglingsalter. Acta morph. hung. *7:* 423 (1956–57); cit. ATERMAN (chap. 3).

GARCÉS, H. y LEIVA, W.: Hepatitis infecciosa congénita en gemelos univitelinos. Revue chil. Pediat. *25:* 427 (1954).

GELLIS, S. S.: Comment to the paper of SCOTT *et al.* Year book of pediatrics, p. 102 (Year Book Med. Publishers, Chicago 1954).

GERMAN, J. L.: Autosomal trisomy of group 16–18 chromosome. J. Pediat. *60:* 503 (1962).

GHERARDI, G. and MACMAHON, H. E.: Hypoplasia of terminal bile ducts. Am. J. Dis. Child. *120:* 151 (1970).

GILLESPIE, A.; DORMAN, D.; WALKER-SMITH, J. A., and YU, J. S.: Neonatal hepatitis and Australia antigen. Lancet *ii: 1081 (1970).*

GLAISTER, J.: Lancet *i:* 293 (1879); cit. SWEET (chap. 2).

GOCKE, D. J. and KANEY, N. B.: Hepatitis antigen. Correlation with disease and infectiosity of blood donors. Lancet *i:* 1055 (1969).

GOULD, A. A.: Boston M. S. J. *53:* 109 (1855); cit. SWEET (chap. 2).

HEROLD, A.: Beitrag zur Ätiologie, pathologischen Anatomie und Pathogenese der kindlichen Leberzirrhose. Helv. paediat. Acta *4:* 427 (1955).

HOPKINS, N. K.: Congenital absence of common bile duct. Three cases in one family. Lancet *61:* 90 (1941).

HSIA, D. Y.; BOGGS, J. D.; DRISCOLL, S., and GELLIS, S. S.: Prolonged obstructive jaundice in infancy. V. Genetic compounds in neonatal hepatitis. Am. J. Dis. Child. *95:* 485 (1958).

JANNEWAY, C. A.: In discussion of STOCKES, WOLMAN, BLANCHARD and FARQUHAR's paper.

JOHNSON, A. M. and ALPER, C.: Deficiency of antitrypsin in childhood liver disease. Pediatrics, Springfield *46:* 921 (1970).

KAJII, T.: Thalidomide experience in Japan. Annls paediat. *205:* 341 (1965).

KAYER, R. and YAKOVAC, W. C.: In contribution to BRENT's paper (chap. 1).

KÖHLER, H., *et al.:* Epist. Com.; cit. APODACA J. (1968).

KRAUS, A. M.: Familial extrahepatic biliary atresia. J. Pediat. *65:* 933 (1964).

KRUGMAN, S.; GILES, J. P., and HAMMOND, J.: Infectious hepatitis. Evidence of two clinical, epidemiological and immunological types of infection. J. Am. med. Ass. *200:* 365 (1967).

KRUGMAN, S. and WARD, R.: Infectious diseases of children, p. 103 (C. V. MOSBY, St. Louis 1964).

LAMY, M. and FRÉZAL, J.: The frequency of congenital malformations. Congenital malformations. Proc. 1st Int. Conf., London 1960, p. 34 (Lippincott, Philadelphia 1961); cit. TÖNDURY.

LAPLANE, R.; GRAVELEAU, D.; LODDS, C. et NOUM, I.: Les hépatities néonatales familiales. Pediatrie *19:* 217 (1964).

LELONG, M.; ALAGILLE, D. et BOUQUIER, J.: Contribution à l'étude de la transmission transplacentaire de l'hépatitie viral. Revue int. Hépat. *8:* 919 (1961).

LELONG, M.; ALAGILLE, D.; LE TAN VINH et WOLF, A.: La cholestase intrahépatique chronique du nourrisson et du jeune enfant. Sem. Hôp. Ann. Ped. *36:* 2271, P/371 (1960).

LONDON, W. T.; SUTNICK, A. I., and BLUMBERG, B. S.: Australia antigen and acute viral hepatitis. Ann intern. Med. *70:* 55 (1969).

MACCALLUM, F. O.: Transmission of arsenotherapy jaundice by blood. Failure with faeces and nasopharyngeal washings. Lancet *i:* 342 (1945).

MACINTOSH, R.; MERRIT, K. K.; RICHARDS, M. K.; SAMUELS, M. H., and BELLOWS, M. T.: Pediatrics, Springfield *14:* 505 (1954); cit. TÖNDURY.

MANSON, M. M.; LONGAN, W. P., and LOY, R. M.: Rubella and other virus infections during pregnancy. Rep. of Publ. Hlth and Med. Subjects, No. 101, p. 1 (1960).

MIETENS, C.: Desarrollo e importancia de las inmunoglobulinas en el lactante. Folia clin. intern. *21:* 10 (1971).

MILLER, B.: Neonatal hepatitis in one of the binovular twins. Am. J. Dis. Child. *94:* 308 (1957).

MIRICK, G. S. and SHANK, R. E.: An epidemic of serum hepatitis. Studies uncontrolled conditions. Trans. Am. clin. climat. Ass. *71:* 176 (1959); cit. KRUGMAN *et al.*

MIRICK, G. S.; WARD, M. D., and McCOLLUM, R. W.: Modification of posttransfusion hepatitis by gammaglobulin. New Engl. J. Med. *273:* 59 (1965).

MUNK, K. und RUNNEBAUM, H.: Virus-Infektionen nach Organtransplantationen bei immunosuppressiver Therapie. Dt. med. Wschr. *95:* 2252 (1970).

NEEFE, J. R.; GELLIS, S. S., and STOCKES, J., jr.: Homologous serum hepatitis and infectious (epidemic) hepatitis. Studies on volunteers bearing on immunological and other characteristics of etiological agents. Am. J. Med. *1:* 3 (1946).

NEEL, I. V.: Am. J. hum. Genet. *10:* 398 (1958); cit. TÖNDURY.

NEWMAN, C. G. H.: Prenatal varicela. Lancet *ii:* 1159 (1965).

PAKTORIS, E. A.: Gamma-globulin in the prophilaxis of epidemic hepatitis. 9th Int. Congr. Microbiology, Moscow 1966, abstr., p. 394.

PERALTA, A.; HUERTAS, H.; CONTRERAS, F. y GRACIA BOUTHELIER, R.: Distress respiratorio del recién nacido por mucoviscidosis con atresia de las vías biliares. Referat. Pediat. 8: 57 (1968).

PÉREZ-SOLER, A. and ESPADALER, J. M.: Ataxia-telangectasia. An. de Medic. Especial. 1: 294 (1964).

PERRIN, D.; GUIMBRETIERE, J. et HAROUSSEAU, H.: Une nouvelle forme d'incompatibilité fœto-maternel: L'hépatite néo-natale familiale. Presse méd. 74: 1307 (1966).

PILLOUD, P.: L'hépatite néo-natale. Méd. Hyg. 24: 230 (1966).

PRETE, S. DEL; CONSTANTINO, D., and DOGLIA, M.: Different Australia antigen determinants in acute viral hepatitis. Lancet ii: 292 (1970a).

PRETE, S. DEL; DOGLIA, M.; ADJUKIEWICZ, A. B.; FOX, R. A.; CONSTANTINO, D.; GRAZIINA, A.; DUDLEY, F. J., and SHERLOCK, S.: Detection of a new serum-antigen in three epidemics of short-incubation hepatitis. Lancet ii: 579 (1970b).

PRINCE, A. M.; HARGRONE, R. L.; SZUMENESE, W.; CHERUBIN, C. E.; FONTANA, V. J., and HEFRIES, G. H.: Immunological distinction between infectious and serum hepatitis. New Engl. J. Med. 282: 987 (1970).

QUICK, A. J.: Sporadic hemophilia. Archs intern. Med. 106: 335 (1960).

ROTH, D. and DUNCAN, P. A.: Primary carcinoma of the liver after giant-cell hepatitis of infancy. Cancer 8: 986 (1955).

SANVALD, R. und SAUERBRUCK, T.: Australia(SH)-Antigen bei Blutspendern und -Empfängern. Dt. med. Wschr. 95: 2153 (1970).

SCHMID, M.: Ikterus in der Schwangerschaft. Dt. med. Wschr. 94: 1332 (1969).

SHARP, H. L.; BRIDGES, R. A.; KRIVIT, W., and FREIER, E. F.: Cirrhosis associated with alpha-1-antitrypsin deficiency: a previously unrecognized inherited disorder. J. Lab. clin. Med. 73: 934 (1969).

SIMMEL, H.: Zentbl. Path. 32: 593 (1921–22); cit. SWEET and KRAUS (chap. 2).

SMITH, D. W.; PATUA, K.; THERMAN, E., and INHORN, S. L.: No. 18 trisomic syndrome. J. Pediat. 60: 513 (1962).

SMITHWICK, M. and GO SUAT CHEN: Hepatitis-associated antigen in cord and maternal sera. Lancet ii: 1081 (1970).

STOCKES, J., jr.; WOLMAN, I. J.; BLANCHARD, M. C., and FARQUHAR, J. D.: Viral hepatitis in the newborn. Clinical features, epidemiology and pathology. Am. J. Dis. Child. 82: 213 (1951).

STOCKES, J., jr.; BERK, J. E.; MALAMUT, L. L.; DRAKE, M. E.; BARONDESS, J. A.; BASHE, W. J.; WOLMAN, I. J.; FARQUHAR, J. D.; BEVAN, B.; DRUMOND, R. J.; MAYCOCK, W. D.; CAPS, R. B., and BENNET, A. M.: The carrier state in viral hepatitis. J. Am. med. Ass. 154: 1059 (1954).

TAYLOR, P. E.; ALMEIDA, J. D.; ZUKERMAN, A. J., and LEACH, J. M.: Relationship of Milan antigen to abnormal serum lipoprotein. Am. J. Dis. Child. 123: 329 (1972).

THALER, M. M.: Fatal neonatal cirrhosis. Entity or end result? A comparative study of 24 cases. Pediatrics, Springfield 33: 721 (1964A).

THALHAMMER, O.: Pränatale Erkrankungen des Menschen, p. 47 ff. (G. Thieme, Stuttgart 1967).

THOMAS, W.: New Zeald med. J. 4: 161 (1891); cit. THOMPSON (chap. 5).

TOLENTINO, P.: Itteroneonatale da atresia delle vie biliari intrahepati che con cellule giganti polinucleate dopo hepatite materna in gravidanza. G. Mal. infett. 11: 1116 (1959).

TOLENTINO, P.; BRAITO, A., and TASSARA, A.: HAA and congenital biliary atresia. Lancet i: 398 (1971).

TÖNDURY, G.: Ätiologische Faktoren bei menschlichen Missbildungen. Triangel, Basel 7: 90 (1965).

WEICHSEL, M. E. and LUZZATTI, L.: Trisomy 17–18 with congenital extrahepatic biliary atresia and congenital amputation of the left foot. J. Pediat. 67: 324 (1965).

WHITTEN, W. W. and ADIE, G.: Congenital biliary atresia. Report of three cases, two occurring in one family. J. Pediat. 40: 539 (1952).

WINDMILLER, J.; MARKS, J. F.; EKKEHARD, W. R.; COSTALES, F., and PEAKE, C.: 17–18 Trisomy with biliary atresia. Report of a case. J. Pediat. 67: 327 (1965).

WOLFF, E.: Etude de 134 mongoliens. Annls paediat. Suppl. 202 (1964).

WONG, P. W. K.; BURNSTINE, R., and HSIA, K. Y.: Neonatal hepatitis in a twin. Pediatrics, Springfield 36: 138 (1965).

ZONDECK, B. and BROMBERG, Y. M.: Infectious hepatitis in pregnancy. J. Mt Sinai Hosp. 14: 222 (1947).

Chapter 7

Other Nosological Aspects of the Inflammatory and Atresia-Inducing Disease

We have described the inflammatory and atresia-inducing disease from a pathogenic point of view, based on the pathological data and its histopathogenesis, as an inflammatory disease with a more or less intense and extensive injury of the liver and bile ducts. The triad, understandably, must present a background with some peculiar characteristics and must have some limits. This background depends on the pathogenic status and the boundaries on the etiological conditions.

Before discussing the subject, some terminological and conceptual questions should be precised.

I. Terminology

The word 'atresia', from 'a' without and 'tresos' hole: lack of lumen, is quite different from other expressions, in particular from 'obstruction' (intrinsic and extrinsic), which means abolition of the lumen by an external cause; in this case the lumen becomes virtual; it does not disappear primarily, but perhaps secondarily.

Nevertheless, the general consensus conceives the term atresia as something more than the simple lack of a lumen. It interprets 'atresia' as an obliteration of the structure which outlines and limits the lumen, i.e. of the epithelial and perhaps any other cover component, in the first and primordial place; complete or partial lengthways, but always total in the transversal sense, even if it only occurs in a small zone. The absence of structure due to a formation defect has a well-established name, agenesia, and its partial defect due to the same cause, hypogenesia. In a similar way, the structure that once formed does not grow will show reduced dimensions and will suffer aplasia or hypoplasia. *Atresia is thus a term reserved to the absence of a structure which, once formed, has been destroyed.*

The term 'atresia' fits very well in the case of absence of real lumen of the excretory structures in extrahepatic atresia; usually there are remnants, at least microscopically visible, of the layers of the organ, especially of the internal one, indicating that the organ existed and later has suffered a deleterious action.

But it is not so proper to talk about intrahepatic atresia, especially of the small portal ducts. In this case, the organ is limited by a simple epithelial layer (because even when surrounded by conjunctive tissue it has the characteristics of a lax adventital one). When this tissue is destroyed, the duct also disappears and as there are no vestiges left of it it is not possible to precise whether it was destroyed or perhaps it was never formed.

It would then be more exact to talk of ductipenia in partial cases and of absence or disappearance in complete cases. Nevertheless, the use of the term atresia is fully justified due to the fact that in the destroyed excretory structures the fundamental fact occurs: disappearance of the lumen.

II. Conceptual Problems

1. Neonatal hepatitis considered within the frame of the triad is defined by a histological image with the following features: (a) Some inflammatory manifestations which are more or less intense with or without transformation of the hepatocytes into giant cells. (b) A certain ductipenia, real or apparent or both. (c) More or less pronounced phenomena of d-d-n of the structures and a reactional dynamic to the injury, with proliferation and d-d-n (proliferation-degeneration).

The sum of real ductipenia (visible or not) and apparent ductipenia lies between 20 and 50%[40].

Such an image does not permit a definitive diagnosis of neonatal hepatitis, but only a provisional one; only the clinical and pathological evolutive course will confirm it, especially when the cholestatic syndrome is practically total: fecal elimination of ^{131}I-rose bengal is less than 10% in 48 h.

2. We consider that a true intrahepatic atresia exists when the real ductipenia, evidenced by the absence of inflammatory reaction, is over 50%.

3. Even in total intrahepatic atresia, it is always possible to observe some normal ducts, or ducts more or less affected by the d-d-n process. It is understandable, on the other hand, that normal ducts, and ducts affected by d-d-n, can only be seen in a good-sized surgical biopsy.

4. Taking into account the evolutive character of the process, it is understandable that the histological examination is not always decisive with regard to atresia,

---

40 Our data are not extensive enough to permit further precision. In this respect, it should be noted that a d-d-n of the epithelium, which could lead to a real ductipenia of small proportions, can be seen in many processes – apart from those indicated in figure 15 – even in hepatic cirrhosis due to mucoviscidosis [VOLEJNIK et al., 1965].

especially at the beginning of the disease; it can even be frankly misleading. It is necessary to be very cautious not to establish a diagnosis that can be erroneous.

5. To obtain pathological information that can be valuable to delineate the state of the excretory structures, it is necessary to observe at least 10 conjunctive spaces, including the Kiernan and septal spaces, which should be easily legible, without artifacts due to handling. Due to the size of the fragment obtained by needle biopsy, it is easy to deduce that on many occasions it will be insufficient to obtain the necessary data.

Let us now consider in detail the special nosological aspects that outline the inflammatory and atresia-inducing disease.

A. Etiological Element

The triad has some limits which depend on a well-defined etiology: Figure 15 shows the close relationship between the three entities and their possible etiological agents.

There is a *primary cause,* acquired postconceptionally, which acts during the fetal period producing a hepatopathy, and that can also act during the embrionary period causing malformations.

a. Infectious Cause

Viral agents. A well-known causal agent in some cases is admitted by many authors: the virus of hepatitis. Other infectious agents are not as often involved as the hepatitis virus. The rubella virus is the causal agent of the inflammatory and atresia-inducing disease in a few cases. It is not known whether other infectious viruses can be considered as etiological factors. The most controversial one is the cytomegaly virus.

The cytomegaly virus has been found in a good number of cases of neonatal hepatitis [WELLER and HANSHAW, 1962, chap. 3; DANKS, 1969, chap. 1] and precisely in 'neonatal hepatitis', i.e. in neonatal hepatitis with giant cell transformation [WELLER and HANSHAW, 1962, chap. 3]. Thus, it should be considered as a possible causal agent, although the number of cases in which it has been found is still small and a superimposed or perhaps basic infection cannot be ruled out.

On the other hand, the cytomegalic virus has rarely been found in cases of atresia.

This possible agent is not mentioned in the extensive review of MEGÉVAND [1963]; it was not found in any of the 10 cases of extrahepatic atresia of WELLER and HANSHAW [1962, chap. 3] and the 20 cases of DANKS [1969, chap. 1]. We know of only three cases of atresia in which features of the cytomegalic disease were found; all of them have peculiar characteristics. In the case of SEIFERT and OEHME

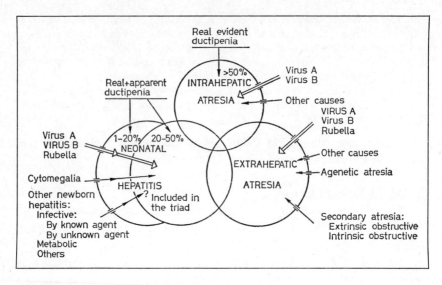

Fig. 15

[1957], classified by the authors as hypoplasy of the bile ducts with hepatic cirrhosis, no cytomegalic cells were found in the liver. The case history included a maternal hepatitis during pregnancy, and a twin sister of the patient also suffered hepatitis. In the case of STERN and TUCKER [1969], multinucleated giant cells, but not cytomegalic ones, were found in the liver. In the case cited by GUBERN-SALISACHS [1968, chap. 5], from PEREZ DEL PULGAR and VILA TORRES, no cytomegalic cells were found in the liver, and the mother lived during pregnancy with two of her sisters affected by infectious hepatitis.

In summary, no evidence exists as of now to affirm that these cases of atresia are due to the cytomegalic virus or whether the infection is superimposed on a process caused by the real etiological virus, which could be such a ubiquitous one as the hepatitis virus. We are inclined to accept the second hypothesis, especially in view of the high frequency of the cytomegalic infection[41] and the very low incidence of discovery of the cytomegalic virus in atresia.

Bacterial agents. The cases in which a bacterial etiology of atresia can be suspected are exceptional. BECROFT [1972] has very recently de-

---

41 10.6% of the cases that died between birth and 1 year of age, according to the data of SEIFERT and OEHME [1957]. This figure was deduced from the 9% given by the authors for children between 0 and 15 years. The cytomegalic infection seldom produces clinical symptoms, as STARR *et al.* [1970] have proved very recently.

scribed one case that could be the result of an infection by Listeria mono-
cytogenes. Since this would be the only case due to listeriosis, this interpretation should be taken with care, as in the case of cytomegalic viruses.

b. Noninfectious Etiology

a) In spite of the fact that *erythroblastosis* has been mentioned as a
possible causal agent of atresia, we believe that the few cases of extrahepatic atresia with erythroblastosis described are merely coincidental, as in
the case of atresia and cytomegalic infection.

Some authors simply dismiss the isoimmunity hypothesis of atresia, suggesting
that the organic biliary plugs cannot be a cause of atresia, because this process appears too early. We do not think that this argument permits the discarding of isoimmunization as a cause of atresia, since as a rule, atresia develops through the late
fetal period and first stages of extrauterine life. The organic plugs, embodiment of
the *classical inspissated bile,* might produce pathological changes of the intrahepatic
ducts, as SHERLOCK [1969, chap. 1] has pointed out, but not in the large ducts,
which are empty due to a process of cholestasis. It is also improbable that the mere
lack of use can produce atresia as it only results in hypothrophy of the excretory
channels. Thus, it seems more logical to suppose that isoimmunization is just a
coincidence and not a true synthropy in the genesis of atresia.

b) Neither can an *abnormal fetal bilirubin* be incriminated in the genesis of atresia. The bilirubin apparently becomes abnormal as a result of
the pathological process, as in all other hepatic disease, but not the other
way around.

In our concept of the inflammatory and atresia-inducing disease, the
cases due to a *secondary cause,* e.g. extrahepatic atresias due to another
well-defined disease from an etiological point of view, must not be properly included in it (fig. 15).

B. Pathogenic Element

The disease show a background in which some characteristics can
be separated, taking into account the two aspects – inflammation and
atresia.

a) On the part of the atresia-inducing component. The background
is well conformed and allows little confusion.

In extrahepatic atresia: The lack of lumen by destruction of the epithelial elements of the organ, inherent to a hepatic-biliary inflammation, is
quite different from the one that can be produced by a secondary cause, intrinsic or extrinsic, in which it is easy to demonstrate the etiology of the obstruction (ring-shaped pancreas, pseudocytes of the common bile duct, etc.).

In intrahepatic atresia: Every case of intrahepatic atresia with clinical signs before three months of age is classified as inflammatory 'atresying' disease, even when the inflammatory component is scarce or missing.

We admit with PILLOUD [1966, chap. 1] that the inflammatory process is not always present, because at the time of the histological observation it may have subsided. As has been reasoned in chapter 5 (pp. 126 ff.), it seems very improbable that a case of intrahepatic atresia can be the expression of aplasia or agenesia. The syndrome of MACMAHON and THANNHAUSER [1952] described as 'congenital dysplasia of the interlobular ducts with extensive cutaneous xanthomatosis' (acholangic congenital biliary cirrhosis) is, in our opinion, a *congenital* intrahepatic biliary atresia, not an aplasic or agenesic disease that needs a long time to develop one of its characteristic symptoms: xanthomatosis. The same pathogenesis is valid in the *acquired* MacMahon-Thannhauser syndrome, which appears in later ages, both in the child and in the adult. The observations of ductipenia recently described by SHARP *et al.* [1967b, chap. 1] some of which had already begun in the neonatal period, are also part of it.

The lack or the minimal appearance of ductipenia permits one to exclude diseases such as congenital hepatic fibrosis, fibroangiomatosis of the bile ducts and neonatal hepatic cirrhosis from the 'atresying' syndrome.

b) On the part of the inflammatory component. The inflammatory background is much less specific, due to the fact that a patent inflammation with giant cells tand trabecular distortion is common to a good number of diseases with a well-defined etiology: syphilis, hemolytic anemia, etc. Even in metabolic diseases like galactosemia and ornithinemia, a histological image coincidental with that of 'neonatal hepatitis' can exist. In these cases, however, the injury to the excretory epithelial structures is missing or is scarce. On the other hand, there are cases of inflammatory and atresia-inducing disease in which such a giant cell transformation and trabecular distorsion are nonexistent.

Conclusion: The inflammatory and atresia-inducing disease is especially centered on the atresia-inducing component and its previous process, the d-d-n of the excretory epithelial structure.

References

BECROFT, D. M. O.: Biliary atresia associated with prenatal infection by *Listeria monocytoegenes*. Archs Dis. Childh. *47:* 656 (1972).

MACMAHON, H. E. and THANNHAUSER, J. J.: Congenital dysplasia of the interlobular bile ducts with extensive skin xanthomatosis. Gastroenterology *21:* 448 (1952).

MEGÉVAND, A.: Embryopathie cérébrale dans un cas de maladie généralisée des inclusions cytomégaliques. Annls paediat. *201:* 410 (1963).

SEIFERT, G. und OEHME, J.: Pathologie und Klinik der Cytomegalie, pp. 22, 57, 72 (Thieme, Leipzig 1957).

STARR, J. G.; BART, R. D., jr., and GOLD, E.: Inapparent congenital cytomegalic virus infection. Clinical and epidemiological characteristics in early infancy. New Engl. J. Med. *282:* 1075 (1970).

STERN, H. and TUCKER, S.: Cytomegalic infection in the newborn and in early childhood. Three atypical cases. Lancet *ii:* 1268 (1969).

VOLEJNIK, J.; DUSEK, J.; BENDA, K. und ROCECK, V.: Die Lebercirrhose bei der Mucoviscidosis. Annls paediat. *204:* 108 (1965).

Chapter 8

Nosological-Therapeutical Advantages of the Unitarian Pathogenic Concept of the Triad

We believe that in considering a case of neonatal jaundice in which, the serum bilirubin levels are higher than 3–5 mg% other causes of predominantly direct, or indirect hyperbilirubinemia have been ruled out, by exclusion, a concept of a unitarian pathogeny will alow a better understanding of the diseases included in it, from the diagnostic, evolutive and therapeutic points of view.

I. With Regard to the Diagnosis

a) If the ^{131}I-rose bengal test shows an elimination higher than 10% after 48 h a well-established extrahepatic biliary atresia may be initially ruled out.

b) If the figure is lower than 10%, the most likely is that we are dealing with a case of extrahepatic atresia. Nevertheless, neither neonatal hepatitis nor intrahepatic atresia may be absolutely ruled out. In this circumstance, a strict follow-up of the case is required to reach a diagnosis, paying special attention to: (1) Repeated determinations of bilirubin and stercobilin content in feces. (2) Repeating the ^{131}I-rose bengal test one month later. A needle biopsy of the liver can be useful. Nevertheless, if carried out precociously, before two months of age, no great value can be attached to it, because: the specimen obtained may be too small, and at this time the histological signs of the disease to be ruled out, i.e. those of extrahepatic atresia, are not usually very prominent.

It is not advisable to perform a surgical exploration before this time.

II. With Regard to the Course

a) The process can resolve itself spontaneously because we are dealing with a case of neonatal hepatitis with a ductal d-d-n component of little intensity, i.e. a hepatic injury that does not endanger the large ducts (or if it does, it has not altered their function). This will occur if the process is of scarce intensity or there is an immunobiological situation that allows to fight with advantage against the morbid noxa; counting on a good capacity of regeneration of the ductal system, the process will end up with a 'restitutio ad integrum', or perhaps with a partial recovery, by development of a scar of fibrous tissue which leads to cirrhosis.

b) Due to a lack of defences, the process could attain a greater intensity, following the path of extrahepatic biliary atresia and/or intrahepatic atresia.

c) Finally, a change in the immunobiological reactivity of the organism, accompanied by an increase in the capacity of regeneration of the extrahepatic ducts, can later condition the formation of epithelial excretory structures which, if not capable of a total recanalization of the initially atresic ducts, at least will allow the performance of a bilio-intestinal anastomosis.

III. With Regard to the Treatment

a) Extrahepatic atresia may be incurable because there is no way to treat it when accompanied by intrahepatic atresia.

b) Cases of exclusively extrahepatic atresia offer a better outlook, especially when a cystic formation in the hepatic hilum is found that would allow an anastomosis.

c) When a cystic formation of this type is not found, the concept that the dynamics of the process permit one to await, in a few cases, a more or less significant regeneration of the atretic ducts, imposes the performance of a hepato-duodenal anastomosis.

Chapter 9

Evolutive Course of the Entities of the Triad in Regard to their Pathology and Treatment

Although in chapter 3 (sect. V), we have discussed the dynamics of the triad in its general features, we believe it important to further consider the subject.

I. Neonatal Hepatitis

The patterns of evolution it may follow are:

a) *Ordinary evolution,* with progressive tendency to healing, which is usually obtained with anatomical and functional restitution. According to our observations, little defects consisting in dysmorphy or atresia of some ducts and moderate fibrosis may remain, perhaps more frequently than one could suppose. Nevertheless, these lesions are compatible with a normal hepatic function (case 9, p. 222).

b) *Malignant evolution,* with hepatic *miopragia* leading to coma. This evolutive form is rare, and seldom mentioned.

c) An evolution towards a predominantly *intrahepatic atresia.* Microscopic examination of successive tissue samples confirm that instead of a progress towards resolution, the d-d-n phenomena of the ductal system becomes progressively more severe.

d) Towards extrahepatic atresia. Perhaps at the time the diagnosis of hepatitis is made the atresia already exists, but the appearance is that of 'hepatitis'.

e) *Healing* (?) with sequelae. (1) With simple fibrosis and with a component of more or less severe ductipenia, with little or no functional disorder, and with limited or absent tendency to progress. (2) With a clear cirrhotic picture, above all in intervened cases, with marked alteration in

function and with an uncertain future although, according to our observations, the treatment with steroids seems to influence it favorably (case
1, p. 213).

STOWENS [1966, chap. 2] in relation with the evolution of neonatal hepatitis
(espeicifically of the giant cells disease) gives the following figures: 40% evolve towards healing – the giant cells disappear, and no sequelae remain; 40% develop fibrosis and cirrhosis of the organ, and in 20%, the disease remains unchanged, the
giant cells *do not regenerate* (the author says) and death occurs at an earlier or later
date.

II. Extrahepatic Atresia

Its evolutive possibilities are as follows:

a) *Biliary cirrhosis secondary to biliary atresia* with increasing atrophy and dysfunction of the parenchyma, leading to a progressive deterioration of the homeostasis before 'stressors', especially infections. The
child usually dies within 6–24 months, although cases of longer survival
have been reported.

b) The performance of anastomosis with efficient recovery of the bile
flow to the gut has been a clear demonstration that the cirrhotic tissue is
not always so irreversible [CAMERON and BUNTON, 1960, chap. 1; THALER
and GELLIS, 1968a–d, chap. 1; KASSAI *et al.*, 1968, chap. 1].

III. Intrahepatic Atresia

Two types of evolution may be observed:

a) *Towards* a more or less evident *fibrosis,* predominantly of the portal spaces. A marked ductipenia is always present at least of 50%, as the
result of the severity of the d-d-n process and of the regeneration capacity
of the ductal system (case 14, p. 227).

It is worth pointing out that even with a marked ductipenia, the excretion of
the pigment tends to be little decreased. The more altered and reduced are the elimination of cholesterol and trioxy and dioxy acids to which we must ascribe, especially to the latter, the greater part of responsibility for the most outstanding symptom
in ductipenia, i.e. itching.

The clinical picture, the laboratory characteristics, and the small sys-
temic and homeostatic alteration, explain why usually this evolutive form
of intrahepatic biliary atresia is compatible with a long survival. What is

especially outstanding is that the bilirubin excretion, as already mentioned, remains hardly altered, and the hyperbilirubinemia is minimal.

Several theories have been offered to explain this. The most accepted one indicates that the retained pigment in the liver is reabsorbed by the lymphatics and catabolized elsewhere. Others think that the production of bile is clearly diminished. To our judgment, the little clinical intensity of the process, in particular from the hyperbilirubinemia point of view, would be specially related to the three following elements: (1) it is known that a small part of the gland is sufficient to carry out all its physiological duties[42]; (2) the bile elimination defect is not total, because a certain number of ducts *always remains,* and (3) the bilirubin that is secreted and cannot be excreted is reabsorbed and passes to the blood to be secreted again, and when repeating this cycle many times there is a moment when it can be excreted because it finds some patent intrahepatic ducts.

b) Apart from this evolution towards hepatic fibrosis, a less frequent but clear *evolution towards cirrhosis m*ay occur, with the characteristic appearance of primary biliary cirrhosis, classically known as hypertrophic cirrhosis of Hanot and also by the more modern denomination cholangiolythic hepatitis, i.e. an inflammatory 'destruction of the interlobar ducts' [BAGGENSTOSS, 1966, chap. 2] or a 'chronic destructive nonsuppurated cholangitis' [RUBIN et al., 1965].

None of our own cases of intrahepatic atresia or those we have been able to review that still survive appear to have shown this picture of primary biliary cirrhosis, but only that of scar fibrosis properly demonstrated in one of them by a surgical hepatic biopsy at the age of 3 years (case 14, p. 227, cpl. XII). But indeed, we have observed this evolutive form in the case of a girl presenting an acquired McMahon-Thannhauser syndrome, which started at the age of $4^1/_2$ months, and who died at the age of 18.

Reference

RUBIN, E.; SHAFFNER, F., and POPPER, H.: Primary biliary cirrhosis. Chronic non-suppurative destructive cholangitis. Am. J. Path. *46:* 387 (1965).

42   According to MCMASTER and ROUS [WITH, 1968, chap. 1] dogs do not show jaundice until 95% of the bile ducts are ligated. RICH's theory [WITH, 1968, chap. 1] is based on this point. If the bilirubin production is normal, only 5% of normal hepatic tissue suffices to avoid hyperbilirubinemia. In a similar way did MANN and BOLLMANN [with 1968, chap. 1] express themselves years ago: only after the extirpation of 70% of the gland does a transitory hyperbilirubinemia occur.

Chapter 10

Surgical Indications

Now we will consider the surgical indications in the triad syndrome, taking into account the intensity of cholestasis and their likely influence on the evolution of hepatitis.

For a long time, when surgical techniques had not reached the present degree of efficiency, authorized voices [SANTULLI et al., 1960; DANKS and BODIAN, 1963, chap. 1] pointed out that it did not seem reasonable to operate on any case of obstructive jaundice, malformative or pseudomalformative, considering the *poor operative risk* to the hepatitis patients. An abdominal intervention with the inherent manipulation of the ductal region, added to the surgical trauma itself, showed little *prospect of success* in saving the life of an unusual case of atresia where an anastomosis of the 'agenesic' rests of the ducts with the intestine could be carried out, whereas there would be many more cases of hepatitis *not* needing any surgery and regrettably terminating by surgical death.

The operatory risk still exists nowadays, but *not* as an early postoperative fatal outcome. *A delayed risk* exists sometimes long after the intervention has been carried out; the danger of hepatic fibrosis-cirrhosis time after the operative act, due to anesthesia or to other causes, has been recently confirmed by THALER and GELLIS [1968 a–d, chap. 1] in a statistically significant series. For these reasons, the operative indication of a case of triad should be carefully weighed and reasoned.

I. Evaluation of the Severity of Bile Retention

a) In the case of complete cholestasis. With absence of bilirubin or stercobilin in the feces, no urobilinuria, and elimination of ^{131}I-rose bengal below 10% after 48 h, we will think as *most likely but not absolutely sure* to be dealing with a case of atresia of the extrahepatic ducts; but an extensive intrahepatic atresia, or a severely cholestatic neonatal hepatitis, must be also considered. Correct information will be obtained by means of a needle biopsy of the liver which can give us a very probable diagnosis of extrahepatic atresia if three elements are found: portal fibrosis, proliferation of the ductal-ductular system, and the presence of bile thrombi within it.

As we know, the last of these features is considered almost as pathognomonic. These three elements are well evident when the process already has been in evolution for some time in extrauterine life.

With such biopsy findings, surgery is fully justified, or rather it is compulsory, aiming to solve the physiopathological disorder. Should it not be due to atresia, another cause of blockade (intrinsic or extrinsic obstruction) also amenable to surgical treatment might be found. If these histological features are not found, further observation and study of the case is in order.

b) In the case of partial or intermittent cholestasis. With constant or transient presence of bilirubin and stercobilin in feces, urobilinuria, and ^{131}I-rose bengal elimination above 10% after 48 h, the diagnoses which may be considered are intrahepatic biliary atresia and neonatal hepatitis.

The needle biopsy will be very valuable if it shows a clear picture of atresia with a marked true ductipenia over 50%. In this case, the patient will be kept under observation and surgery is not indicated.

Nevertheless, if no improvement takes place within a period of 3–5 months, perhaps some benefit may be obtained from a surgical drainage of the gallbladder, in order to insure a greater pressure gradient between the bile ducts and the external space.

II. Evaluation of the Surgical and Delayed Risks

Both the surgical and delayed risks must be considered. The surgical risk is related to the general condition of the patient, to the severity of the disease, to possible nutritional disturbances, etc. *The delayed risks* are not directly related to the operative act (p. 197).

When the clinical picture, laboratory data, hepatic function tests (especially the ^{131}I-rose bengal) and the needle biopsy of the liver do not conclusively support the diagnosis of extrahepatic blockage, the operation should be delayed, until the age of 4–5 months, a time when the cases of hepatitis have developed a full-blown symptomatology or have already reached a significant degree of involution, and the distinction between the diseases requiring an exclusively medical treatment from the ones which can be improved through surgery becomes easy.

Waiting all this time will ensure us against the danger of determining an evolution towards cirrhosis, in a case of intervened hepatitis. On the other hand, if we are dealing with a case of extrahepatic atresia which might be surgically corrected, the fibrosis produced up to them will not be probably irreversible, according to CAMERON and BUNTON [1960, chap. 1], THALER and GELLIS [1968a–d, chap. 1], and KASSAI *et al.* [1968, chap. 1], as mentioned in section I.

Reference

SANTULLI, T. V.; HARRIS, R. C., and REMSTOWA, K.: Surgical exploration of obstructive jaundice in infancy. Pediatrics, Springfield *26:* 27 (1960).

Chapter 11

Treatment

I. Exploratory Timing

The fundamental aim of the explorations undertaken, and the therapy indicated in a case which may correspond to one of the entities of the triad, is centered on the need to *demonstrate extrahepatic atresia* as early as possible, so that the changes of success of the intervention are most favorable.

1. *Divergent opinions have been sustained* concerning the most convenient moment of the intervention. In view of the different conceptions, especially evolutive, of atresia and hepatitis, and the perspectives of success of the surgical intervention in atresia, different indications have been given concerning the most favorable moment for the surgical exploration to reach a diagnosis and especially to try to restore biliary drainage in the case of extrahepatic atresia.

a) Initially, no fixed criteria existed until the general preference seemed to be to operate rather late; at the 4th month or even later, as surgical mortality is high in intrahepatic disease and the exploration of infants is difficult due to the small size of the structures [HARRIS *et al.*, 1954]. BENNET [1964, chap. 1] recommended waiting until the age of 3 months or even later if a tendency to a decrease in serum bilirubin levels is observed.

b) Later on, the opinions became more favorable to advise the operation before the age of 3 months, between the second and the third, so that a secondary biliary cirrhosis which at this time would probably be irreversible has not yet developed.

The opinion of some authors [GELLIS, 1965–66] has varied from advocating surgery between the first and the third month to waiting for 4 months.

c) Nowadays, at *a third stage, two somewhat divergent opinions* are being held: (1) THALER and GELLIS [1968a–d, chap. 1] taking into account the bad prognosis of the cases of hepatitis that underwent a surgical exploration, frequently developing a chronic hepatopathy, and very often a cirrhosis, recommend to operate at about the fourth month but not before, once the evolution has helped to reach a diagnosis, and because up to that moment the fibrotic element has only attained a moderate growth. The operated cases of atresia in which an anastomosis could be performed demonstrate that the fibrotic-cirrhotic process developed up to that date is not fatally irreversible. (2) KASSAI *et al.* [1968, chap. 1], who have treated with success cases of extrahepatic atresia by means of a hepatoenterostomy, recommend that the operation should be carried out before 3 months of age, because their satisfactory results had been observed in cases operated upon before this date.

II. Two-and-a-Half-Month Plan

Two-and-half months after the jaundice first appears, a diagnostic conclusion should be reached to either accept or discard an extrahepatic atresia. In the present state of our knowledge, the most convenient method of study of the patient to determine the possible need of surgical therapy is as follows:

A. First Month
Weekly or every 10 days: Carry out blood, feces and urine examinations to discard: (a) icteric disease with indirect hyperbilirubinemia – hemolytic diseases of the newborn; Crigler-Najjar syndrome; etc., and (b) other diseases with direct hyperbilirubinemia – septic infections; cytomegaly; etc.

B. Second Month
Continue the examinations, every 2 weeks or even more frequently.

Between 4 and 6 weeks, if there are no signs that the ducts are about to open, cholestasis does not decrease clearly, and especially if bilirubin and/or stercobilin in the feces remain negative, one should resort to: exploration with ^{131}I-rose bengal and hepatic needle biopsy.

An elimination below 10% after 48 h will indicate that the parenchyma is very much affected or that an extrahepatic atresia exists.

Even when elimination is moderately above 10%, atresia cannot be categorically discarded, due to the rather infrequent fact that it may have not yet completely developed.

A needle biopsy will be valuable, not to show a definite entity of the triad, as it is too soon for the histological picture of extrahepatic atresia to have developed, but to eliminate other types of jaundice with direct hyperbilirubinemia, such as Dubin-Johnson's, Rotor's and Summerskill and Walsche's diseases, etc.

C. Middle of the Third Month

If the data of blood, feces and urine examinations continue to be little explicit, the ^{131}I-rose bengal test[43] should be repeated; if a high figure (beyond 15–20%), which would indicate an obvious 'opening' of the ducts is not obtained, the needle biopsy should be repeated. The corre-

43 A double dose of ^{131}I-rose bengal will fall in the margin of good tolerance, because according to GHADIMI and SASS-KORTSAK [1961, chap. 1], a 1-min fluoroscopy will expose the patient to a radioactivity which is 90 times higher for the whole body, 9 times for the liver and 13 times higher for the gonads than that produced by a simple rose bengal test.

Recently, RAINER POLEY et al. [1972, chap. 1] have combined the ^{131}I-rose bengal test with cholestyramine. This cationic binding resin should inhibit the enterohepatic cycle of the rose bengal, thus increasing its elimination by the stools in cases of hepatitis; this increased elimination can be proved in vitro, by simulating the bowel conditions. The authors have used this combined rose bengal-cholestyramine test in 18 children, 1–6 months old, with a prolonged jaundice that they subdivide into 3 groups. Group A includes 10 children with extrahepatic biliary obstruction, confirmed during the intervention; in all cases lipoprotein X was positive. Group B included 5 children with intrahepatic cholestasis with a moderate increase of serum total bilirubin (>9 mg%); in 3 of them the lipoprotein X was positive, and in the other 2 it was negatve. In group C, with moderate cholestasis, lipoprotein X was negative and the figure of ^{131}I-rose bengal elimination was compatible with a patency of the external ducts. In the group A patients with a mean excretion of the labeled product of 5% (range 1.9%) at 96 h, cholestyramine increased it to 7% (range 3–9%). In the patients of group B with neonatal hepatitis and a mean elimination of 5% (range 3–7%) without cholestyramine, the fecal elimination increased to a mean of 23% (range 13–36%) after cholestyramine.

Very recently, CAMPBELL et al. [1974] have shown that the serum levels of lipoprotein X decrease after a 2-week treatment with cholestyramine (4 g per day) in cases of neonatal hepatitis, whereas they actually increase in cases of atresia. Should these observations be confirmed, the differential diagnosis of hepatitis and atresia would become surprisingly simplified.

Table XI. Correlation between laboratory data, diagnosis, and surgical therapy

Rose bengal test	Needle biopsy	Diagnosis	Surgery
A. Very low elimination[1]	hepatic signs of extra atresia[2]	extra atresia *without* intra	yes
B. Very low elimination[1]	no hepatic signs of extra atresia; only intra	extra and intra atresia	no, because it is ineffective
C. Low elimination[3]	image of intra atresia similar or more marked than in the first exploration	intra atresia[4]	no
D. Lower elimination than in the first exploration	more marked signs of intra atresia	hepatitis developing into intra atresia	no
E. Elimination similar or higher than in the first exploration	same injuries or improved image	hepatitis without developing into intra atresia	no
F. Lower elimination than in the first exploration with a figure of extra atresia	more intense injuries of hepatitis	possible extra atresia	yes? better to repeat spec. expl. at 4 months; if they show the same result, intervention

1 Within the figures for extra hepatic atresia: below 10% after 48 h [THALER and GELLIS, 1968a–d, chap. 1].
2 Signs of portal fibrosis, ductal-ductular proliferation and on many occasions bile thrombi, mainly in the ducts, but less frequently than in a surgical biopsy due to the smaller size of the specimen.
3 Fluctuating around the figure of extra hepatic atresia.
4 Can be confused with the previous one if the rose bengal elimination is very low. As it does not require intervention, the diagnosis has no practical value as far as surgery is concerned.

lation between these explorations, the admissible diagnosis, and the therapeutical behavior are included in table XI.

Summing up: One should not wait more than 3 months to operate a case in which a diagnosis of extrahepatic atresia is reached with the indicated study methods or in which extrahepatic atresia is highly suspected, especially in view of the results of a liver biopsy showing signs of external blockade. The fact that a longer delay will result in more dilations of the deteriorated ducts [DANKS et al., 1968, chap. 2], does not preclude a greater surgical success; on the other hand, the best results of a hepatoenterostomy are obtained before this date [KASSAI et al., 1968, chap. 1].

The best results of an intervention can be expected in group A (table XI) where signs of regeneration-proliferation of the ducts exist. They will be worst in group F, where a 'hepatitis' is correlated with only moderate or even scarce regeneration-proliferation of the excretory element. Finally, the possibilities of cure or even improvement are nil in group B.

III. Limitations to the Efficiency of the 'Two-and-a-Half-Month Plan'

A. By Defect

1. *Gentle or very slow evolution of the process.* The pathological picture will not have acquired a definite, sufficiently expressive image. Cases of such a nature are not infrequent. Only considering that a definite diagnosis ['ultimate diagnosis' of HAYS et al., 1967, chap. 1] is not made until after a long time, will we have an easy explanation to this contingency which can be encountered during the diagnosis of an entity belonging to the 'inflammatory and atresia-inducing disease' and will provoke the anxiety of clinicians and pathologists on certain occasions.

How should one proceed in this eventuality? In a hepatopathy which reveals no indication of aperture of the ducts in a period of $2^1/_2$–3 months (case F of fig. 4) and *in which the histological signs are not clearly expressive of extrahepatic atresia,* we believe that the best attitude is to wait until the age of 4 months and repeat the special explorations. If the result is not conclusive, repair to the intervention.

This is better carried out in two operative sessions. In the first session, a cholangiography and a surgical hepatic biopsy, which will permit a study on a larger part of gland are performed. If it is demonstrated that the ducts are not normal and the histological study shows an image corresponding not to hepatitis but to atresia, we will try to resolve the biliary blockage in a second session. Thus, the infant will not be exposed to a long exploration which might be dangerous.

2. In some unusual cases, such as 'erroneous' cases (p. 62), a histological image of hepatitis may be accompanied by extrahepatic atresia.

The number of such cases, which in our opinion are mixed cases, and clearly explainable within the concept of inflammatory and atresia-inducing disease according to the literature on the subject, seems to be certainly small but not negligible.

A further limitation by defect, not corresponding to the triad, may be the case of an external blockage due to an extrinsic or intrinsic obstructive cause, whose hepatic histological image is that of a hepatitis, instead of the usual extrahepatic atresia. These cases are easy to explain on the basis of the previous paragraphs in this section. A simple obstruction does not necessarily imply a lesion of the ducts. On the other hand, they are easily diagnosed using other clinical-radiological methods.

B. By Excess

To operate a case of hepatitis because it is believed to correspond to extrahepatic atresia cannot be considered as a limitation by excess. Taking into account that usually a histological image of hepatitis corresponds to hepatitis if the case is intervened, the excess will only be ... on the surgeon's decision.

Nevertheless, it is possible to ask: can there really be a *limit by excess* to the efficiency of the '$2^1/_2$-month plan'? We believe not.

However, it is possible that a hepatic image of extrahepatic atresia would correspond to a case with some normal external ducts, but in which the operative cholangiography does not offer a normal image of the large intrahepatic duct near the hilum, i.e. we will be confronted with a case of extra-intrahepatic atresia. And this, as is understandable, does not imply a limitation to the efficiency of the plan that we propose.

IV. Surgical Treatment and its Perspectives of Success

A. Extrahepatic Atresia
1. To Restore the Bile Flow
Anastomosis of the remnants of large external ducts or of the hilum to the intestine. LADD [1928] was the first to perform a successful operation in a case of extrahepatic atresia. Since then, a great amount of work has been published on the surgical treatment of atresia. The published reports point out an operability which fluctuates between 4 and 50% [SILVERBERG et al., 1960, chap. 1].

HASSE [1965] has studied the structure of the normal liver on the newborn in 40 cases and indicated that the resection of the quadrate lobe can show the existence of a hepatic duct with a blind end that could be useful to establish an anastomosis, but usually this duct is too small. The ducts in the periphery of the juxtahilar system are also small in size and do not permit a bile derivation. Only the hepatic duct itself is of a suitable dimension to reestablish a functional bile flow.

Recently, RIGHINI [1969] has indicated that at present more than 80% of the patients with biliary atresia reveal anomalies of such a kind that cannot be corrected and the treatments employed are totally or partly useless. ROMUALDI *et al.* [1969], with similar views, indicate that the type of atresia in which there is a dilation of the hepatic duct, through an atresia of the common bile duct, is the only one that can be surgically corrected.

At present, it seems that the search for a dilatation in the deteriorated ducts or near them to perform an anastomosis is facilitated by the exploration, previous to the laparotomy, by means of ultrasonic echography. According to SURUGA *et al.* [1969, chap. 2], this physical method permits to detect the presence of dilated remains of the intrahepatic ducts.
One can also evidence with this exploratory procedure the dilatation of the common bile duct through a cyst[44] even when it is small. The ultrasonic echo even detects fine and pointed echos which proceed from the interior of the gland in cases of cirrhosis; on the contrary, in cases of hepatitis the hepatic tissue appears as homogeneous as a normal liver. These data offer good perspectives for the differential diagnosis of the triad and the diagnosis of atresia and hepatitis.

In the statistics of GROSS [1953, chap. 1], including 146 cases, an operable anomaly was found in 18% of them, but the bile flow was successfully reestabished in only 8%[45]. The statistics of KASSAI *et al.* [1968, chap. 1] show similar figures. In 81 cases (deducting 6 from the total number, 87, because they were due to a ductal obstruction by a common bile duct cyst [46]) 14 were liable to surgical correction, which was successful in only a few cases.

2. Other Procedures to Restore the Liver-Intestine Bile Flow
Drainage of the liver by means of Sterling-Southey tubes. The results obtained with this method have been practically useless. WELTE [1971, chap. 3] has recently confirmed this prediction.

44 The difficult cases (i.e. those that show jaundice without a tumor or abdominal pain) can be evidenced before the intervention. That is to say that a precocious diagnosis, which will make surgical correction possible before an irreversible cirrhosis has become evident, can be performed.
45 These data emphasize how different are operability and clinical cure (p. 72).
46 Atresia of the corresponding segment of the common bile duct is secondary to an inflammatory process due to the retention of bile as the result of an anomaly of the duct [BABBIT, 1969].

Hepatoenterostomy. This operation, recommended by LONGMIRE and SANFORD [1946 and 1949], was proved useful by SILVERBERG *et al.* [1960, chap. 1]. At present, the hepatoenterostomy operation permits the resolution of some cases of extrahepatic atresia in which an anastomosis between the remnants of ducts and the intestine is not feasible especially using the technique of KASSAI *et al.* [1968, chap. 1].

In 53 cases of extrahepatic atresia considered surgically incorrectable (without a remnant of hepatic duct or a bag that would allow a derivation) and in which a hepato-enterostomy was practiced, 20 showed an excellent or good secretion and 6 cured completely between 14 months and 13 years after the operation. In all but one of them, the laboratory examinations are almost normal. In 6 cases, a hepatic needle biopsy showed a nearly total recovery of the parenchyma, with disappearance of the fibrosis and cholestasis. In relation to the perspectives of success of the hepatoenterostomy, the following points should be taken into account:

a) The rate of success improves when the bile ducts found in the histological examination of the hilum (of the porta hepatis) are larger than 200 nm. In 10 out of 14 cases with ducts of this size, a good postoperative bile excretion was obtained, while it was only obtained in one out of 13 cases with ducts of less than 150 nm.

b) All cured cases were operated before the age of 4 months.

c) According to KASSAI *et al.* [1968, chap. 1], the clinical and histological experience has clearly demonstrated that many cases with ducts of the porta hepatis larger than 200 nm can be cured if they are operated before that age, and preferably during the first 3 months after birth.

Nevertheless, the results obtained by the Japanese authors have not been confirmed by CAMPBELL *et al.* [1974]. These authors have treated 9 cases of extrahepatic biliary atresia (incorrectable type) with hepatic portoenterostomy. All showed unremitting progression of biliary cirrhosis (as documented by regular postoperative percutaneous liver biopsies and autopsy examinations) and no evidence of improved bile secretion. Survival statistics for this group of infants reveal that their survival time is actually worse than that reported for patients with untreated biliary atresia. This study raises serious questions regarding the efficacy of hepatic portoenterostomy in the treatment of extrahepatic biliary atresia.

Certainly, the results reported by KASSAI *et al.* [1968, chap. 1] and CAMPBELL *et al.* [1974] are widely dissimilar. How can this be explained?

Assuming in the authors a similar level of surgical performance (similar technique, comparable technical skills, etc.), the better results reported by the Japanese authors could be explained accepting that their cases are less severe; it could well be that the d-d-n process in the excretory structures was less marked and with a slighter component of intrahepatic atresia, and allowed a better regeneration at the level of the anastomosis, preserving its patency. In a way, this would be the opinion of CAMPBELL [1974], when he states: 'The Japanese are operating on a different entity.' In our opinion, it would probably be better to speak of a qualitatively different form of atresia.

Reintervention. On some occasions [KANOF *et al.*, 1953, chap. 3; DE-LAITRE *et al.*, 1960], a second intervention, practiced several months after the first, permitted the discovery of a dilated biliary structure amenable to be anastomosed.

Recently, DUHAMEL [1969] has reintervened three cases which initially had presented no anastomosable ducts, but in which the biopsy suggested that one should wait for juxtahiliar biliary dilatation of the intrahepatic ducts. In two of them, the dissection of the hilum revealed a blind formation with which a derivation was practiced. One of the two recovered.

3. Derivation of the Bile Excretion by Means of Lymphatic Drainage

The opening of the great lymphatic trunk into the esophagus is an operation that has been employed by ABSOLON *et al.* [1965] and SURUGA *et al.* [1965]. The experience with this heroic procedure is small, but the results obtained so far are not hopeful.

The scarce perspectives of success seem to depend more on the maintenance of the drainage than on technical difficulties of the intervention. The lymphatic drainage operation is offered as the only perspective of possible success in the treatment of coetaneous intrahepatic and extrahepatic atresia.

B. Intrahepatic Atresia

With the surgical intervention, it is pretended to establish a greater pressure gradient between the liver and the rate of excretion; this should logically take place by communicating the bile ducts with the exterior. This procedure, however, has not proved efficient, as ALAGILLE *et al.* [1969, chap. 1] indicate.

The chelant treatment of the bile-acid excretion by cholestyramine shows more favorable perspectives (p. 209).

V. Other Therapeutic Measures that Can Be Beneficial in the Treatment of the Triad

These are all symptomatic, unspecific measures, because there is no etiological treatment.

First, because an etiology based on the hepatitis virus has not been really demonstrated, a second because even if it were the causal agent, no anti-infectious or
semispecific means are available at present.

A. Dietetic Treatment

Immediate principles, minerals and vitamins. According to the needs
of the patient, proteins and carbohydrates will be administered and there
is no reason to establish a limitation of the lipidic contribution, except
when lipids are not tolerated.

If they produce dyspepsia, they can be made more tolerable by the administration of biled preparations or by limiting their intake to half (use of semidefatted
milk).

The mineral and vitamin administration will have to be complete to
cover the developmental demands. Liposoluble vitamins, especially A
and D will be administered in a hydrosoluble fashion.

B. Medical Treatment

Cholagogues and choleretics. One can expect no beneficial result
from them.

Hepatic protectors. Nucleosides of the pyrimidine type, uridine, and
cytidine seem especially recommendable, to reintegrate RNA to the
hepatic cell and activate the biosynthesis of lipotropic factors (lecithins),
influencing favorably the carbohydrate metabolism, etc.

Corticosteroids. Glycocorticoids. Their value is scarce in neonatal
hepatitis and viral hepatitis of children and adults. However, a certain fe-
vorable action can be expected due to their anti-inflammatory action, and
they can be administered during brief periods. For example, 15 days of
treatment and another 15 days or a month of rest. At the beginning, using
a dose of attack and later on decreasing gradually: 3 days at 3 mg/kg/day;
4 days at 2 mg/kg/day; and 8 days at 1 mg/kg/day.

The treatment is combined with antibiotic protection, at moderate
or small doses.

Cholestyramine. This is a product that combines with the bile acids
both *in vitro* and *in vivo,* preventing their reabsorption. Used at important doses and over a certain period of time, a patent decrease in retained
bile acids is obtained, and their figures in blood decrease to normal levels.
With this, a patent improvement of the pruritus is obtained.

Other altered biological constants, such as bilirubinemia and BSP also improve;
the high figures of phosphatemia are not influenced. Sometimes, a moderate

alteration of sleep during the night indicates that the process, although improved, continues.

When the treatment is long, the growth process [SHARP et al., 1967b, chap. 1], which is always notably retarded, reassumes its normal rhythm. The dosage has to be high. For a child of 5–6 years, about 15 g, daily [SHARP et al., 1967a, chap. 1]. In consequence, for infants we use doses of 2–3 g per day. With the administration of such doses, no secondary effects have been observed. Only after 1 or 2 months, a notable beneficial effect is observed. This is explained because the 'pool' of bile acids of the organism is important and takes time to be moved.

Enhancement of bilirubin conjugation and its catabolism. In this sense it may be useful in certain cases to apply phototherapy and the administration of uridin-diphospho-glucose, phenobarbital, etc.

VI. New Therapeutic Perspectives

Liver transplant. According to CHAPUIS [1969], the ideal indication of the liver transplant is, without any doubt, atresia of the bile ducts in the child. It seems this is the only solution for the mixed cases of extrahepatic and intrahepatic atresia which are the most frequent ones, as has already been shown in detail (p. 58). WILLIAMS [1970] has practiced it in a case of atresia without survival.

Very recently, LILLY and STARZL [1974, chap. 1] published a very remarkable contribution to the treatment of biliary atresia by means of orthotopic transplantation of the liver. These authors report significantly long survivals in a number of their 29 cases thus treated, with one of the patients surviving for over $4^1/_3$ years.

The encouraging results achieved by STARZL's group add more interest to a continued research to improve the results of the treatment of biliary atresia.

Perhaps another possibility of treatment would be the graft of a healthy liver fragment [ELIAS, 1967, chap. 5]. We are dealing here also with a transplant, which is partial, but probably subject to the same contingencies as a total transplant.

References

ABSOLON, K. B.; RICKERS, H., and AUST, J. B.: Thoracic duct lymph drainage in congenital biliary atresia. Surgery Gynec. Obstet. *120:* 123 (1965).

BABBIT, D. P.: Congenital choledochal cyst. New etiological concept based on anomalous relationships of the common bile duct and pancreatic duct. Ann. Radiol. *12:* 231 (1969).

CAMPBELL, D.: in Discussion on the paper of CAMPBELL, RAINER POLEY, ALAUPOVIC and IDE SMITH The differential diagnosis of neonatal hepatitis and biliary atresia. J. Pediat. Surg. *9:* 699 (1974).

CAMPBELL, D. P.; RAINER POLEY, J.; BÄHTIA, M., and IDE SMITH, E.: Hepatic portoenterostomy: is it indicated in the treatment of biliary atresia? J. pediat. Surg. *9:* 329 (1974).

CHAPUIS, Y.: Transplantation hépatique chez l'homme. Premiers resultats. Perspectives d'avenir. Presse méd. *77:* 203 (1969).

DELAITRE; PERTUS; VARLET et PERRIN: Atrésie complète des voies biliaires réopérée tardivement. Archs fr. Pédiat. *17:* 674 (1960).

DUHAMEL, B.: Ictères congénitaux. Riv. Chir. pediat. *11:* 251 (1969).

GELLIS, S. S.: Comment to Bennet's paper; cit. Yb. Pediat., p. 186 (Chicago 1965–66 series).

HARRIS, R. C.; ANDERSEN, D. H., and DAY, R. L.: Obstructive jaundice in infants with normal biliary tree. Pediatrics, Springfield *13:* 293 (1954).

HASSE, W.: Intrahepatic vascular and bile-duct systems as related to operative treatment of bile-duct atresia. Archs Dis. Childh. *40:* 162 (1965).

LADD, W. E.: Congenital atresia and stenosis of the bile ducts. J. Am. med. Ass. *7:* 1082 (1928).

LONGMIRE, W. P., jr. and SANFORD, M. D.: Intrahepatic Cholangiojejunostomy with partial hepatectomy for biliary obstruction. Surgery, St Louis *24:* 264 (1946).

LONGMIRE, W. P., jr. and SANFORD, M. C.: Further studies. Ann. Surg. *130:* 458 (1949).

RIGHINI, A.: L'atresia congenita delle vie biliari. Esperienza in 18 casi. Riv. Chir. pediat. *11:* 255 (1969).

ROMUALDI, P.; BERGAMI, F. e ROMUALDI, C.: Sulla chirurgia del fegato e delle ipertensione portale nel bambino. Riv. Chir. pediat. *11:* 267 (1969).

SURUGA, K.; YAMAZAKI, Z.; IWAY, S.; NAGASHIMA, K., and WORI, W.: The surgery of infantile obstructive jaundice. Archs Dis. Childh. *40:* 158 (1965).

WILLIAMS, R.: Transplantation of the liver in man. Br. med. J. *i:* 585 (1970).

Chapter 12

Prophylaxis of the Diseases of the Triad

Until recently, no measure could be taken in this sense. However, considering the very probable hepatitic viral etiology for a great number of cases, a ray of light seems to illuminate the dark field of inoperance. CZAPO et al. [1964] have recently obtained favorable results in their attempts to prevent epidemic hepatitis in children by means of an alcohol-attenuated virus obtained from adult patients' serum, and with the addition of γ-globulin. KRUGMAN et al. [1971] have obtained good results in the preventive treatment of homologue serum hepatitis by means of boiled serum from hepatitis patients.

References

CZAPO, J.; NIERGES, G.; BUDAL, J.; LICHTEN, P., and TOTH, I.: Experiments with attenuated epidemic hepatitis virus. Annls paediat. *202:* 72 (1964).
KRUGMAN, S.; GILES, J. P., and HAMMOND, J.: Viral hepatitis: type B (MS-2 strain). Studies on active immunization. J. Am. med. Ass. *217:* 41 (1971).

Appendix

Summarized Description of the Cases Mentioned in the Text

Case 1

L. B. V., a 2-month-old infant, was born on 3-17-1962, the product of a normal, full-term pregnancy. His birth weight was 3,950 g. Meconium, normal. Breast-fed. 24 h after birth, a patent jaundice, which became more marked during the following days, was observed; with yellowish feces, and an increasingly choluric urine. Three days after birth, a blood analysis yielded the following data: total bilirubinemia, 17.37 mg%, of which 4.1 mg% corresponded to direct bilirubin.

This clinical picture was still present when he was seen by us at the age of 2 months.

Physical examination showed a markedly hypotrophic child, with a weight of only 4,400 g.

Good general condition. The liver and spleen were palpable 5 and 2.5 cm below the costal margins.

Laboratory data

Morphological: Erythrocytes, 3,700,000/mm³; Hb, 68%; leukocytes, 12,500/mm³. Leukocytic formula: segmented, 25%; juvenile, 4%; lymphocytes, 58%; monocytes, 11%, and eosinophils, 2%; reticulocytes, 20‰.

Blood groups: B, Rh, positive; Coombs, negative.

Chemistry: Bilirubinemia, total, 10.32 mg%, of which 5.32 mg% direct. Transaminases: GO, 73 U; GP, 42 U; alkaline phosphatase, 22 Bodansky (B) U.

The jaundice continued to increase, to the point that a week later (5-24-62) the feces had become completely acholic, although once in a while greenish mucous masses were excreted, sometimes in large amounts; no bilirubin or stercobilin were found in them. The transaminases increased markedly: GO, 296 U, and GP, 92 U; cholesterol, 1.8 g%.

By this time, the liver reached the right iliac fossa over the inguinal fold; the spleen also increased in size (5½ cm). As a result, a surgical exploration was recommended, and carried out at the age of 3 months (6-20-72). Laparotomy revealed visible bile ducts with a small amount of greenish-whitish bile in the gallbladder, a large, smooth liver, wine-red in color, and slightly yellowish. Histological examination of a liver biopsy gave the image of a 'classical neonatal hepatitis' with a very intense portitis, abundantly infiltrated by leukocytes and with clear signs of d-d-n in the excretory system, especially at the level of the ducts (cpl. IA, VIIA).

Evolution: A corticosteroid therapy was prescribed. Prednisone 3 mg/kg/day for 5 days; 2 mg/kg/day for 10 days, and 1 mg/kg/day for another 15 days. A few days later, a clear decrease of the liver and spleen size was noted, with a marked improvement in the nutritional state.

15 days after the corticosteroid therapy, the stools became colored and bilirubin-positive again.

On 10-3-62, the jaundice had completely disappeared, the feces were pigmented (stercobilin-positive) and there were no pigments in the urine.

On 12-18-62 the liver and spleen were only 3 and 2 cm below the costal margins.

At 13 months of age, his weight and height were normal; the child already walked and had started to talk.

Nevertheless, the hepatic colloidal lability tests (mesenchymal test) were abnormal with a positive Hanger test $(+++)$ and a Weltmann of 8. Blood proteins were within normal limits: total proteins, 7.89%; albumin, 73%; α_1, 1%; α_2, 7%; β, 6%, and γ, 13%.

Two months later, and in spite of his good general condition, *the spleen enlarged markedly* to 5 cm below the costal margin.

In spite of an intense corticosteroid therapy (like the first one, but prolonged for 15 more days) the spleen remained enlarged, 3 months later reaching 6 cm. The blood tests showed a slight hypersplenism, especially on the platelet side (130,000/mm³) and a marked granulocytopenia.

At the age of 2 years, and in spite of different liver-protecting treatments (hepatic extracts, orotic acid, etc.) the spleen size had not changed, and remained at the same level. The liver, however, had decreased noticeably to 2 cm.

At the age of 3 years; the general condition was good. Spleen unmodified.

Blood: Alkaline phosphatase, 9.5 BU; transaminases, GO, 12; GP, 15 BU; prothrombin time, 80%. These results suggest that the mesenchymal hyperplasia of the liver and the spleen, i.e. the hepatic cirrhosis, is slight, as the protein tests did not demonstrate a hypergammaglobulinemia.

At the age of 4 years, the good general condition was maintained. The state of the splenoportal circulation was determined by means of a transparietal splenoportography, which showed a sinuosity and moderate dilation of the splenic vein; a normal portal vein, and very marked intrahepatic ramification, especially of the small vessels, which take a long time to empty, demonstrating a certain difficulty in the passage of blood through the parenchyma. There were no visible collateral vessels. The manometric pressures were not determined, because the conditions in which they are carried out (anesthesia, apnea) make them very doubtful.

At the age of 4¹/₂ years, the patient was treated with 6-mercaptopurine at a dose of 2 mg/kg/day which was carried out for nearly 2 years, with regular interruptions to allow for 15-day prednisone treatments. During this time, the size of the liver and spleen remained unchanged. The child's development was normal in every aspect; weight at the age of 6, 19,700 g. However, he still showed some signs of hyperesplenism: anemia of 3,500,000/mm³ and leukopenia of 2,800/mm³; platelets were normal. Nevertheless, there are no ostensible humoral signs of clear hepatic cirrhosis: Blood proteins, total, 6.9 g⁰/o. Electrophoresis, albumin, 55⁰/o; α_1, 2⁰/o; α_2, 6⁰/o; β, 18⁰/o, and γ, 19⁰/o. A hepatic *needle biopsy* only showed a slight portal fibrosis. In some of the Kiernan's spaces the ducts were apparently missing (without any histological changes in the hepatocytes), but this could not be determined with certainty.

For 1¹/₂ years, he continued in good general condition, with no limitation of the activities of his age group. At 8 years of age, his weight was 23,100 g and his height was 1.24 m. A routine check-up yielded the following results:

Erythrocytes, 4,400,000/mm³; Hb, 88⁰/o; leukocytes, 4,700/mm³. Leukocytic formula, segmented, 59⁰/o; eosinophils, 4⁰/o; lymphocytes, 32⁰/o, and monocytes, 5⁰/o; reticulocytes, 2⁰/o.

Blood proteins: Total, 6.8⁰/o; electrophoresis, albumin, 58⁰/o; α_1, 4⁰/o; α_2, 12⁰/o; β, 17⁰/o; γ, 28⁰/o. Transaminases: GO, 52 U, and GP, 12 U. Hanger and cadmium tests, negative; Kunkel, 7 U; MacLagan, 6.7 U.; Weltmann, 6; Takata, negative.

At 8¹/₂ years of age, his general condition was good with a slightly enlarged liver (1.5 cm under the costal margin), and a spleen 1.5 cm below the umbilical level (12 cm from the margin), showing a hard consistency. Once in a while, he was treated with hepatoprotectors (orotic acid and nucleosides). A new control needle biopsy of the liver demonstrated that in some Kiernan's spaces the duct was missing, but this sign could not be properly quantified.

The results of a determination of antigens and antibodies related to viral hepatitis are mentioned in the text (p. 163).

A new observation at the age of nearly 11 years (2-14-73) showed no variation in his residual hypertrophied spleen; but the liver was diminished in size (or perhaps it had moved cranially?) with its border being found by palpation at the level of the costal margin. A psoriasis of slight intensity appears intermittently. A very recent control (11-26-74) has shown the boy to be in good clinical condition, in spite of his large spleen. The pertinent laboratory data are: Transaminases, GO, 20 U; GP, 25 U; alkaline, phosphatase, 6 BU. Proteins, total, 70 g‰. Albumin, 45.24 g‰; globulins, total, 24.76‰; α_1, 1.98‰; α_2, 5.62‰; β, 6.6‰; γ, 10.56‰. Lipids, total, 495 mg⁰/o; cholesterol esterified, 1.45 g‰; free, 0.60‰; triglicerides, 0.95‰, and free fatty acids, 0.14‰. α_1-antitrypsin, 275 mg⁰/o.

Case 2[47]

E. T. G., a 3-month-old girl, born at term on 1-6-1968; a small amount of normal meconium was noted. From the fourth day of life, the feces became clearly acholic, and at the same time a marked choluria became apparent. The total retention jaundice syndrome did not show any changes during the next 3 months. The girl showed a remarkably normal development, but was markedly icteric and pre-

47   This case has been published by GUBERN-SALISACHS, L.; ESCUDÉ CASALS, M. et GUBERN PI, L.: Cas démonstratif de l'origine cicatricielle de l'atrésie des voies biliaires extrahépatiques. Ann. Chir. Infant. *11:* 297 (1970).

sented an hepatomegaly reaching the navel. Before surgery the laboratory data were as follows:

Blood: Total bilirubinemia, $150 \text{ mg}\%_{00}$; autocatalyzed, $135 \text{ mg}\%_{00}$; indirect, $15 \text{ mg}\%_{00}$. Transaminases: GO, 310 U; GP, 500 U. Erythrocytes, $4,000,000/\text{mm}^3$. Leukocytic formula: segmented, 45%; lymphocytes, 54%; monocytes, 1%. Total proteins, 72.10‰; albumin, 34.80‰; $\alpha_1 + \alpha_2$, 13.1‰; β, 7.2‰; γ, 17‰.

Feces: Stercobilin, negative.

A laparotomy demonstrated the presence of a rudimentary gallbladder with hardly any white contents. It was not possible to pass any contrast material through it. At the hepatic-common bile duct junction, acystic cavity with a small quantity of bilious liquid was found, coninued upwards by a fibrous cord. Eight days after surgery, the icteric syndrome remained unmodified; total bilirubinemia 17.7 mg%; of which 10 mg% corresponded to direct bilirubin. The patient died on the 11th day. The necropsy examination revealed very obvious signs of a destructive process of the external ducts (fig. 7, 8) with a characteristic hepatic image of extrahepatic atresia. The fibrous cord that corresponds to the hepatic duct gave the image shown in figure 16.

The sclerolipomatous reaction of the adventitia in the affected organs bears witness to the long duration of the process (fig. 17).

Case 3

M. M. H. G., a 2-month-old girl, born at term on February 3, 1965, weighing 4,000 g. Colored meconium; breast-fed. About the 20th day of life, a marked jaundice was observed, although the date of commencement cannot be fixed with precision. The feces remained colored for some time, turning clearly acholic after about $1^1/_2$ months.

Physical examination: Girl with a relatively good general condition. Her weight progress has been poor: she weighs 4,630 g. Obvious icteric pigmentation on all surfaces of the skin and conjunctives. Hepatomegaly of 6 cm; no splenomegaly. Total direct bilirubinemia, 9.15 mg%. Transaminases: GO, 46 U; GP 48 U. Urine: bile pigments, positive (+++); bile salts positive, (+). The presence of urinary urobilin was demonstrated in three successive analyses.

The process did not improve with treatment. As a result, a laparotomy was indicated at the age of 3 months. It revealed the presence of atrophic ducts, with a rudimentary gallbladder. A hepatic biopsy showed the presence of a ducto-ductular proliferation with very marked conjunctive-portal fibrosis and with signs of biliorrhagia in the connective tissue and phagocytosis of pigments by migrating elements.

The process remained unchanged during the first 8 postoperative days, when the patient died of an acute respiratory process.

This observation does not allow one to establish either a definite or an absolutely sure diagnosis of extrahepatic atresia (autopsy permit was not granted). However, the clinical and surgical data and those derived from the biopsy, with great fibrotic and ductal-ductular proliferation, duct and ductule bile thrombi and signs of biliorrhagia in the connective tissue, and the absence of either extrinsic or intrinsic

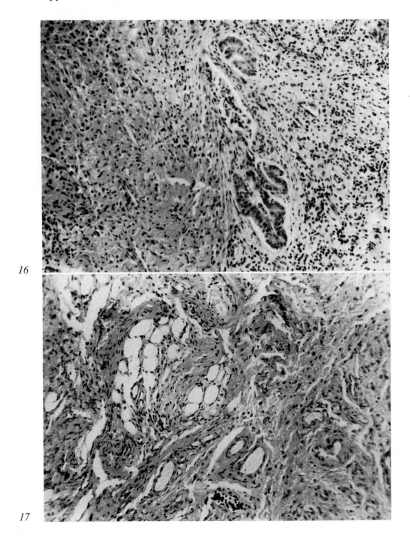

Fig. 16. Hepatic duct, with the aspect of a fibrous cord. To the right, masses of altered muscular tissue. The left connective tissue with dense mononuclear infiltration in which 3 fairly well-preserved epithelial tubes are found, and another one with marked necrobiosis.

Fig. 17. Sclerolipomatous tissue with several delated blood vessels, capillaries and veins, and scarce, diffuse leukocytic infiltration of the mononuclear type.

obstructive cause in the main bile ducts, led us to accept without hesitation the diagnosis of extrahepatic atresia.

Case 4

M. J. A. G., a 55-day-old girl, born at term on 2-19-1965. Colored meconium, bottle-fed. At the end of the second day of life, she presented jaundice, which soon increased. The first stools that followed the passing of meconium were already clearly acholic; soon a patent choluria also appeared.

On the 12th day of life, urine and feces examinations indicated the retentive character of the jaundice: the urine contained pigments but was negative for urobilin; in the feces, indications of bilirubin, with negative stercobilin were found. Repeated examinations at 5 weeks of age gave the same result. She had slight hepatomegaly and splenomegaly. At this age, bilirubinemia was 5.3 mg%, all of it direct, and the transaminases were: GO, 180 U; GP, 130 U. Alkaline phosphatase, 22 BU.

A laparatomy was carried out at 55 days of age. Only remnants of a hardened gallbladder were found, from which no fluid could be obtained by puncture. A catheter was left in it and after 7 days, the injection of contrast material showed the vestiges of a cavity and a small portion of the cystic duct.

A few days after surgery, she passed stools with greenish mucosities, but the feces did not contain bilirubin, which was investigated by the usual Triboulet and Hymans van der Bergh tests.

The jaundice continued, and the girl died at the age of 5 months due to a febrile process, complicated by pneumonia that lasted over 2 weeks.

A *surgical biopsy* showed the presence of bile thrombi in the ducts and a very outstanding fibrous proliferation of the connective tissue, in spite of the short period of extrauterine evolution (55 days), with clear signs of ductal hyperplastic proliferation that acquired a papilliferous character in some zones (cpl. XIVA).

This case deserves a commentary similar to the previous one, with the characteristic feature of a marked ductal-ductular proliferation in spite of the early age.

Case 5

J. C. C., a 3-month-old boy, born at term on 12-3-1966, weighing 3,700 g. Colored meconium, breast-fed. At the age of 15 days, a light icteric pigmentation was noted, accompanied by a patent choluria. Feces were usually almost colorless, but occasionally normal (?), depositions were also passed. Laboratory examinations carried out at the age of $1^{1}/_{2}$ months yielded the following data:

Bilirubinemia: Total, 5.2 mg%; direct, 2.65 mg%; indirect, 2.55 mg%. Pyruvic transaminase, 130 U. Urine: pigments and bile salts, positive. At the age of $2^{1}/_{2}$ months: bilirubinemia, total, 4.65 mg%, of which 3.15 mg% was direct and 1.50 mg% was indirect; pyruvic transaminase, 250 U.

At the time of his admission, the physical examination showed a relatively good nutritional condition, with hepatomegaly of 6 cm and a spleen pole of 4 cm.

Blood: Total bilirubinemia, 16.66 U%, of which 6.83 U% was direct and 9.83 U% was indirect. Alkaline phosphatase, 23 BU. Transaminases: GO, 260 U; GP, 286 U. Urine: bile pigments, slightly positive; urobilin, positive. Marked hypoprothrombinemia, which fluctuated around 40%, was hardly modified during the following days in spite of treatment with high doses of vitamin K and two blood transfusions. An extensive facial hematoma was attributed to it.

In the days following his admittance, the feces became totally acholic and a blood examination showed:

Bilirubinemia: Total, 23.3 U%, of which 15.7 U% was direct and 7.6 U% was indirect. Urine: Bile pigments, positive; urobilin, slightly positive.

At the age of $3^{1}/_{2}$ months, 15 days after his admission, a laparotomy was carried out. The liver showed a yellowy-greenish color with a smooth surface and some bile ducts with a normal morphology but reduced in size. The injection of contrast material showed a normal biliary tree, easily reaching the duodenum; even the ramifications of the hepatic duct filled up easily.

A *hepatic biopsy* revealed a very marked tubular transformation of the parenchyma with slight inflammatory phenomena, especially in the portal spaces. The duct was missing in many of Kiernan's spaces (cpl. III).

The *postoperative course* showed no ostensible change in the icteric syndrome. The only thing worth mentioning is that the urine urobilinogen and urobilin became clearly positive.

Six days after surgery, the child presented a diarrheic syndrome with great dehydration against which all therapy was ineffective; he became extremely adynamic and died very rapidly.

Case 6

J. B. S., a 3-month-old boy, born at term on 7-4-1964, weighing 3.500 g. Breast-fed only a few days. On the third or fourth day, the parents noticed that the feces were acholic and the urine clearly pigmented. On the 15th day, the child had become markedly icteric. Diagnosed of a hepatitis in the rural region where he lived, the child followed different medical treatments, which did not influence his jaundice, acholia and choluria. With this syndrome he was admitted to the Instituto Policlínico of Barcelona on 11-12-1964. At the time of admission the physical examination showed: child with a moderate dystrophy, slight icteric pigmentation, and a hepatomegaly of 4.5 cm.

Blood: Bilirubinemia, 10 mg%, 8 mg% of which corresponded to the immediate kind, and 2 mg% to the retarded kind.

Erythrocytes: 4,400,000/mm³; Hb, 85%; leukocytes, 15,000/mm³; platelets, 390,000/mm³. With the following Rovatti agglutinogram[48], with 100 isolated platelets, there appear: 18 groups of 2 platelets; 8 groups of 3 platelets; 3 groups of 4

48 The normal figures, according to GUASCH's experience, are groups of: 2 platelets, 33 ($\pm$2); 3 platelets, 13 ($\pm$2); 4 platelets, 8 ($\pm$2). Groups of 5 or more platelets can be found, but this is unusual.

platelets; 6 groups of 5 platelets; 8 groups of 6 or more platelets. Proteins, 7.40%, of which 89% were serines. Transaminases: GO, 500 U; GP, 1,200 U.

Urine: Bile pigments, positive (+ +); urobilin, positive.

Feces: Bilirubin, negative; stercobilin, negative.

Four days after his admission, a laparotomy was carried out, revealing a large liver; the hepatic hilum was visualized with difficulty. At this level, but very deeply, two medium-sized ganglia and some membranous remnants which seemed to correspond to an atrophic gallbladder were found. The hepatic artery and the portal vein were identified, but not the hepatic or common bile ducts. A hepatic biopsy showed, in different fields, all three entities of the triad (fig. 6).

Nine days after surgery, an abdominal wall rupture occurred along the incision. The hepatic hilium showed no visible biliorrhagia.

Five days after the rupture, a new one appeared, and 7 days later a third one accompanied by an intestinal ileus due to intestinal adherences. The general condition deteriorated considerably in the course of these accidents and the child died in an atrepsic state.

Case 7

M. P. M. T., a girl, was 4 months old when first observed on 11-4-61. She had been born at term, with a weight of 3,300 g. Meconium? Breast-fed. In the first days of life the girl showed jaundice, the urine was constantly pigmented and the feces decolored although they were occasionally yellowish or greenish.

At the time of admittance (University Pediatric Clinic of Zaragoza) the girl showd a moderate malnutrition (weight 5,500 g) with a rubi-verdinic pigmentation and with a hepatomegaly of 7 cm without splenomegaly. No pruritus was present. The laboratory examinations showed:

Blood: Bilirubinemia, 2.7 mg% of which 1.5 mg% corresponded to the direct type and 1.2 mg% to the indirect. Alkaline phosphatase, 6.5 BU. Transaminases: GO, 320 U; GP, 1,500 U. Cholesterine, 2.96 g%$_{00}$.

Urine: Bile pigments, + + + (on one occasion negative?). Urobilinogen, urobilin, and bile salts, negative.

Feces: Do not contain bilirubin or stercobilin.

Laparotomy: Carried out at the age of 4$^{1}/_{2}$ months. The liver had a cirrhotic aspect, dark color and a hard consistency; slight ascites. The external bile ducts had a normal aspect, although they were reduced in size. The infection of contrast demonstrated the permeability of the gallbladder, common bile and hepatic ducts, the latter filling up to its first ramification. These results suggested the presence of a blockage of the large intrahepatic bile ducts.

A wedge of liver tissue and a medium-sized ganglion found near the hilum were excised for histological examination with the following results:

Liver

Histological image of extrahepatic atresia with extensive portal fibrosis and neoformation of bile ducts. The ducts of the septal spaces showed obvious signs of a d-d-n process. Marked lobular cholestasis and many bile thrombi, especially in the newly formed channels (cpl. IV, VA, XIII).

Ganglion (Apparently Normal)
Postoperative course: During the 40 days following surgery the girl showed no change in her cholestatic icteric syndrome. After being home for a month, she underwent a severe disease, which was not well-defined clinically, and died.

From a biological point of view, it was determined that the bilirubinemia had decreased somewhat (to 2.3 mg^0/o) and that it was mostly indirect (1.9 mg^0/o).

Case 8

M. M., girl born at term on 5-2-1962, with a weight of 3,600 g. Normal meconium. A few hours after birth, multiple petachiae over all the surface of the body were observed. Progressive jaundice and pigmented urine which acquired a remarkable intensity in the course of five days. Hepatomegaly of 5 cm. During this time the feces became almost colorless. Spleen is also hyperplasic, 3 cm below the costal margin.

Laboratory Examinations
Blood: Bilirubinemia (in mg^0/o) – on the second day of life 12.5, of which 12 corresponded to the direct kind. On the third day, 14.5 (14 direct); on the fourth day, 19 (18 direct); on the fifth day, 20 (19.7 direct).

Other examinations carried out during this period of time: Transaminases: GO, 260 U; GP, 1,088 U. Alkaline phosphatase, 22 BU. Blood count: second day – erythrocytes, 3,540,000/mm^3; leukocytes, 38,400/mm^3, and platelets, 54,200/mm^3. On the fifth day – erythrocytes, 3,860,000/mm^3; leukocytes, 21,000/mm^3, and platelets, 120,000/mm^3. Normal hemograms.

Coombs, negative. Coagulation, normal. Hemocultive, negative. Wessermann, negative. No inclusion bodies were found in urine. There is no galactosuria. Sabin-Feldmann, negative. Blood proteins, normal. Mielogram, with very few megakaryocytes.

Bearing in mind the possibility of an obstructive cholestatic jaundice of external origin due to the great preponderance of direct bilirubin, a laparotomy was performed revealing bile ducts without any extrinsic obstruction and not dilated. The injection of serum into the gallbladder gave the feeling of having to overcome an obstacle; the injection produced a moderate dilation of the common bile duct, which also offered a certain difficulty to the passage of liquid, easily overcome.

The lack of dilation of the ducts invalidates these obstacles as being the cause of an exclusive or preponderant blockage of bile circulation, and the physiopathology of the increase of direct blood bilirubin should be explained by some other mechanism than a simple obstruction. The *histological study* of a hepatic wedge revealed an image of neonatal hepatitis with a moderate amount of giant cells, and a very intense lobular cholestasis, especially parenchymal. Acute inflammatory phenomena were very intense (cpl. VI, XIIB; fig. 9).

Evolution: Three days after laparotomy, the jaundice rapidly decreased, as did hypocholia, and the urine became progressively clearer. 15 days later, the clinical signs had disappeared and the analytic picture was practically normal. A later control at the age of 7 months confirmed, once again, the cure of the disease.

Case 9

A. G. S., a 13-week-old boy, born on 10-7-1969 after an 8-month pregnancy with a weight of 2,350 g. Normal meconium. The mother had an hepatitis at the age of 11. At 15 days of age he suffered a viral process with moderate diarrhea. He recovered, but had a relapse a few days later with a dehydration syndrome; he was admitted to a hospital and improved rapidly.

A few days later, at the age of $2^1/_2$ months, he showed an icteric syndrome with marked, albeit not intense pigmentation of the skin and conjunctives, choluria and acholic feces. He was seen by us when the syndrome was at its peak, or had perhaps started to decline.

The boy was slightly dystrophic (weight 3,750 g) with a liver of 3.5 cm and a spleen pole of 1.5 cm.

Laboratory Examinations

Blood: Erythrocytes, 3,200,000/mm³; Hb, 56%. Leukocytes, 15.000/mm³. Formula: segmented, 66%; juvenile, 11%; eosinophils, 2%; lymphocytes, 18%; monocytes, 2%. Platelets, 300,000/mm³. Bilirubin: total, 2 mg%; conjugated, 1.2mg%; not conjugated, 0.8 mg%. Transaminases: GO, 40 U; GP, 15 U. Proteins: total, 5.8‰. Albumin/globulin ratio, 41/17.

Urine: Bile pigments, + +; urobilin, + + +. No cytomegalic inclusions were found.

Feces: Stercobilin, +.

Hepatic needle biopsy showed the image of an acute hepatitis with moderate lobular cholestasis and intense inflammation of the interlobular conjunctive spaces. Very marked edema and leukocytic infiltration. The ductipenia (pseudoductipenia?) was so remarkable that it was only possible to recognize some bile ducts, with a very patent dysmorphy-dystrophy (cpl. VIII).

The process followed a favorable course, and choluria disappeared within 15 days.

A control biopsy obtained 5 months later revealed the absence of inflammatory infiltration, and a practically normal texture of the ductal-ductular system, although some ducts showed dysmorphic aspect and small bile granules were seen in some hepatocytes. One month later, the child looked normal (weight 9,000 g at 9 months of age) but a laboratory examination showed that the liver function was not completely normal, as indicated by:

Bilirubinemia: total, 0.8 mg%; not conjugated, 0.5 mg%; conjugated, 0.3 mg%. Transaminases: GO, 50 U; GP, 20 U. Alkaline phosphatase, 22 BU. Thymol and cadmium, negative; Weltmann, 7. Proteins: total, 82 g‰. Albumin/globulin ratio, 40/42. Electrophoresis: α_1, 4.7 g‰; α_2, 11.3‰; β, 12.4‰, and γ, 13.6‰.

At 19 months of age, laboratory examinations were normal.

Case 10

E. M. D., a 2-month-old boy born at term on 7-26-1968, weighing 3,200 g. Normal meconium. At 15 days of age, a yellow pigmentation of the conjunctives, followed quickly by a frankly choluric urine, and depigmented feces became apparent.

At the age of 5 weeks, a urine examination revealed: bile pigments, $+++$; bile salts, $+++$, and urobilin, $+++$.

At 7 weeks, a urine examination showed the same results. Other laboratory data included:

Blood: Moderate anemia (3,440,000/mm³). Total bilirubinemia, 13.5 mg%; of which 9.5 mg% correspond to the direct type. GP Transaminase, 84 U; MacLagan, 4 TU. Alkaline phosphatase, 21 BU.

At 9 weeks of age, it was possible to demonstrate a retentive icteric syndrome with moderate dystrophy. Moderate hepatomegaly of 3 cm. Hypospadias and cryptorchydia; both testes were palpable, although they did not reach the bottom of the scrotum.

Laparotomy: Dark greenish liver, without cirrhotic aspect. No extrahepatic bile ducts are observed; only a very atrophic gallbladder that does not permit a cholangiogram. A hepatic biopsy revealed an inflammatory process that affected mainly the portal spaces with a marked dilation, edema and slight leukocytic infiltration; obvious connective proliferation with fibers widely separated by a serous infiltration. Marked ductipenia. No proliferation of the ducts; neither the ducts nor the ductules show any regeneration; on the contrary, the d-d-n process, especially the latter was very intense (cpl. IXA). Intrahepatic atresia, then, which is being progressively added to an extrahepatic atresia.

Postoperative course: Good postoperative course. The icteric syndrome, nevertheless, remained without variation.

A month after the intervention, the laboratory data were:

Blood: Light anemia, with 3,840,000 erythrocytes/mm³. Bilirubinemia of 15.5 mg%, with 11 mg% of the direct kind; MacLagan, 40 U. Alkaline phosphatase, 14.4 BU. Transaminases: GO, 240 U; GP, 200 U.

Urine: Bile pigments, $++++$; bile salts, $++++$; urobilin, $++++$ (!).

He lived for another 1¹/₂ months and died of an undefined immediate cause.

Neither a definitive nor an absolutely sure diagnosis could be established in this case, but we think that a disease with such a frank d-d-n process and marked ductipenia could only be combined intrahepatic and extrahepatic atresia.

Case 11

A. P. U., a girl born on 4-3-1961. Medical control from birth; daughter of a pediatrician.

Three healthy elder brothers; the mother had a 2-month miscarriage during her third pregnancy, attributed to uterine retroversion. She had a viral 'flu' process when 2¹/₂ months pregnant, which also affected the three children.

Born at term and somewhat hypotrophic; weight, 2,700 g; height, 46 cm. Meconium normal in color and expulsion time; bottle-fed.

At 2 days of age, golden yellow stools. Ten days later, she became frankly acholic, with jaundice of the conjunctives, bile pigments in the urine, and feces showing only vestiges of bilirubin. Bilirubinemia, 5.2 mg%, all direct. Cholestinemia, 1.30 g%.

At 18 days, pigments in the urine increased remarkably.

At one month, intensively jaundiced. Traces of urobilin appeared in the urine. Transaminases: GO, 100 U; GP, 100 U. Cholesterine, 4.8 g‰; alkaline phosphatase, 22 BU.

At $1^1/_2$ months: Total bilirubinemia, 14 mg%, of which 8 mg% indirect. Transaminases: GO, 200 U; GP, 350 U. Moderate hepatomegaly and splenomegaly.

At 7 weeks of age, exploratory laparotomy of the bile ducts and hepatic biopsy. A collapsed gallbladder was found, but its size was actually normal as it was easily distended by a serum injection that did not reach the common bile or hepatic ducts. The aspirated serum was green and the injection of contrast material did not reach farther than the cystic duct. The extrahepatic ducts are fine to the touch and had a certain consistency. These data suggest to the surgeon an extrahepatic atresia, in spite of the fact that the gallbladder was easily distended to a normal size, containing green bile. The clinical evolution confirmed the patency of the bile ducts (see below). How, then, are we to explain why the radiopaque material did not go beyond the cystic duct? It is possible that at the beginning there was a true atresia and that, at a later time, recanalization of the bile ducts occurred or, maybe, some excretion or exudate simply obturated the cystic-main bile duct junction; or, last but not least, there was a technical defect in the surgical exploration.

A hepatic biopsy revealed a typical aspect of intrahepatic atresia, especially of the small septal ducts; in some zones, ductular proliferation was observed (cpl. XIB, XIIA).

The operative findings suggested extrahepatic atresia. However, two observations invalidate this conclusion: (1) during the postoperative days, the girl had some yellow stools, which soon became acholic again, and (2) later in the course of the disease, a marked depigmentation occurred, to the extent that only a slight conjunctival jaundice remained.

Evolution: The girl followed the clinical course of a typical MacMahon-Thannhauser syndrome: with practically constant pruritus (which appeared towards the third month), injuries due to scratching and a constantly high cholesterinemia, which decreased with time; from 6.1 g‰ at the age of $2^1/_2$ months to 3.43 g‰ at the age of 6 years and 8 months (once in a while it was even lower, 3 g‰). The fact that it is not accompanied by xanthomata may be explained by the moderate levels of cholesterinemia.

Towards the age of 6 years, she had recovered almost completely without any form of therapy. Her total bilirubinemia was 0.4 mg%; no pigments in the urine. However, she suffered an almost constant itching (cholesterinemia, 3.32 $g^0/_{00}$; slightly high transaminases, GO, 90 U; GP, 36 U) and presence of bile salts in urine.

At the age of 6 years and 8 months, the physical examination showed a moderately dystrophic status with a weight of 15,900 g, a height of 104.5 cm, a discreet jaundice, and sometimes a very intense pruritus. The laboratory tests showed: Bilirubinemia, total, 1.15 $mg^0/_{00}$, of which 0.65 $mg^0/_{00}$ was direct. Transaminases: GO,

34 U; GP, 23 U. Cholesterol, 3.43 g‰. Normal blood proteins, with a γ-globulin figure somewhat below normal (10%) and negative colloidal lability reactions.

She showed practically the same clinical and biological picture at the age of 10 years (2-4-71). On various occasions, the administration of cholestyramine was attempted, but the girl tolerated it very badly and it had to be suspended.

Case 12

M. P. M. A., a girl born on 1-24-1963. Mother had frequent and repeated vomiting during the whole pregnancy. Born at term. Weight, 3,000 g. Meconium not well-colored. Born with intense cyanosis from which she did not totally recover; a moderate cyanosis remains.

Jaundice and choluria from the second day of life. Up to the 26th day of life, the feces were colored, but later they became definitely acholic. At 19 days of life, the bilirubinemia was 15 mg%, all of it direct.

At the age of 1 month, she showed a frank dystrophy with signs which corresponded to a retention jaundice, and a hepatomegaly of 2.5 cm, without splenomegaly. Marked muscular laxity and signs of cyanotic congenital cardiopathy which, according to the radiological and electrocardiographical data, is diagnosed as Fallot's tetralogy.

In the acme of the retention jaundice syndrome, the direct character of the hyperbilirubinemia was confirmed, but on one occasion an abundant urobilinuria was found (!).

At 40 days of age, a laparotomy was performed, with the following result:

Empty, small gallbladder. The introduction of contrast does not reach beyond it. For this reason, the operatory exploration is continued up to the hilum. An empty common bile duct which continues upwards until it divides into the cystic and hepatic ducts is individualized; dissection of the hepatic duct is continued until it divides in the hilum. None of these ducts seem to be more consistent than usual, but they were neither dilated nor did they contain any bile. The fact that the radiopaque material did not go beyond the cystic duct supports the idea of an extrahepatic atresia, especially because the gallbladder was rudimentary, indistensible, and without green bile. Case 15 is similar to this one. The acholia and jaundice persisted with no changes up to the patient's death.

The clinical and surgical data suggested an external and perhaps an internal atresia, confirmed by a surgical biopsy which revealed an extensive ductipenia which affected both the primary and secondary bile ducts. The few ducts remaining showed signs of atrophy and necrobiosis over a background of amoderate inflammation, without fibrosis.

As hepatitis was histologically discarded, the image of the cholangiography probably corresponded to an extrahepatic atresia; maybe not completely established a few days before, as a urine test still revealed an intense urobilinuria. This concept is upheld by the postoperative course.

Postoperative course: It carried on with an icteric syndrome constant acholia, a cyanotic cardiopathy, and marked dystrophy, until the girl died suddenly 5 months later. Epicritically, this case is similar to case 10.

Case 13

C. E. F., a 40-day-old girl, born at term on 6-2-1964, with a weight of 3,900 g. Urine-like meconium, breast-fed. At birth, she was already jaundiced. Stools acholic from the beginning; the urine was choluric from its first emission. The tests practiced a few hours after birth allowed us to discard isoimmunization and revealed a direct bilirubinemia of 8 mg%; 14 days later, it showed a lower figure, 3.85 mg%, but still with a clear preponderance of the direct kind (3.1 mg%). Two urine tests demonstrate the presence of bile pigments, and in the one practiced at 8 days of age, urobilin was slightly positive.

She was admitted to the hospital at the age of 40 days with an icteric syndrome which had hardly had any unfavorable influence on the trophic state. At this moment, the laboratory examinations showed:

Blood: Erythrocytes, 2,000,000/mm^3; Hb, 45%. Reticulocytes, 25%$_{00}$. Leukocytes, 12,300/mm^3. Leukocytes: neutrophils, 25%; eosinophils, 1%; lymphocytes, 69%; monocytes, 5%. Very abundant and remarkably aglutinated platelets. Transaminases: GO, 90 U; GP, 80 U. Alkaline phosphatase, 24 BU.

Preoperatively, the anemia was corrected by the administration of blood.

She was laparatomized at the age of 47 days. No vestiges of the bile ducts were found, except for a small stump of the gallbladder through which a fine plastic catheter was introduced and that did not admit the injection of any amount of saline; no fluid could be obtained by aspiration. The catheter was left, nevertheless, fixed *in situ*. A wedge biopsy of liver showed a typical image of external hepatic blockage with biliorrhages in the interlobular conjunctive spaces. Pronounced proliferation, especially of the ducts and marked fibrosis.

Postoperative course: No trace of bile could be obtained through the drainage tube; due to this it was removed 7 days later. The operative wound healed quickly and well.

A new blood examination carried out 9 days after the intervention revealed: Erythrocytes, 3,300,000/mm^3; reticulocytes, 15%$_{00}$. Platelets: 720,000/mm^3; with the corresponding Rovatti agglutinogram (normal figures are given in case 6): 29 groups of 2 platelets; 23 groups of 3 platelets; 10 groups of 4 platelets; 11 groups of 5 platelets, and 12 groups of 6 or more platelets[49].

The girl continued with her total retention icteric syndrome and with a moderate dystrophy. When the girl was 8 months old (weight 7,100 g) a new surgical intervention was performed. The liver now showed an even more marked cirrhotic aspect and not even the gallbladder stump was found. The search for a bile excretory dilation in the hilum of the liver or its surroundings which would allow an anastomosis was negative.

Three days after the intervention, she died of a collapse, at least partly attributable to the hepatic miopragia. Epicritically, this case is analogous to case 3.

49   Lipidemia was not determined, so it cannot be asserted whether such a pronounced thrombocytosis resulted from it.

Case 14[50]

A. A., 1 3-year-old girl, born at term. Colored meconium; breast-fed for 2 months. At 15 days of age, an increasingly obvious jaundice appeared. The feces which followed the meconium were acholic (milk-like and soft). Pigmented urine.

At 5 months of age, the yellow color of the skin and conjunctives frankly decreased; nevertheless, a certain subicterus remained. No obvious pruritus was noted until after the age of 1 year.

The physical examination revealed a girl with a marked hypodevelopment: weight, 9,700 g; height, 81 cm. Skin and conjunctives, slightly icteric. She did not present xanthomata. Liver: 1 cm under the costal margin; spleen not enlarged. Separated yellowish teeth with marked irregularities of the enamel.

Laboratory Examinations

Blood: Bilirubinemia, 2.9 mg%, of which 2.7 mg% correspond to the direct type. Transaminases: GO, 30 U; GP, 22 U. Alkaline phosphatase, 26 KU.

Urine: Bile pigments, positive; bile salts, slightly positive; urobiline, positive.

Feces: Stercobilinogen, positive.

Three attempts to obtain bile from the duodenal fluid were negative.

The i.v. injection of contrast allowed the visualization of the gallbladder and the emptying of its contents was achieved after a second attempt with a fatty meal.

The *laparotomy* showed a liver of normal aspect and the cholangiography demonstrated the clear permeability of the external bile ducts. Hepatic biopsy: typical image of intrahepatic atresia. No vestiges of ducts or ductules were observed. Moderate fibrosis with hyalinization of the portal connective (fig. 10).

Ulterior Course

1. At the age of 3 years 3 months, she continued with a syndrome of moderate bilirubinic pigmentation. The pruritus also continued. Blood: total lipids, 8 g%$_{00}$; cholesterol, 1.89 %$_{00}$.

2. At 5 years: She continued with the pruritus and the icteric syndrome practically unmodified.

Case 15

Girl, C. G. M., 2 months 10 days old, born at term on 2-5-1971. She had two healthy brothers, 5 and 4 years old, of a eutocic delivery. Weight 3,140 g. Meconium, normal. No physiological jaundice. Breast-fed during the first month.

Cholic stools during the first 15 days which became frankly acholic after the first month. Choluria and moderate icteric pigmentation at 3 weeks of age which increased until the age of $1\frac{1}{2}$ months. During the last 15 days before we saw her, the feces had been on some occasions yellow-greenish.

At 1 month of age, a blood examination revealed a normal cell picture. Bilirubinemia, 6 mg%, totally direct.

50 Summing up of the observatiotn of M. CARBONELL ESTRANY, included in *Prolonged jaundice in the newborn,* Bulletin of the Catalan Society of Pediatrics, *26:* 424 (1965).

At $1^1/_2$ months: Bilirubinemia of 7 mg, also totally direct. Transaminases: GO, 215 U; GP, 243 U. Alkaline phosphatase, 14 BU. Urine: Bile pigments, ++; bile salts, ++; urobilin, +.

Our observations, on 6-14-1971, showed the following clinical picture of the girl:

Moderately dystrophic, weight 3,800 g with generalized icteric pigmentation, preferently in trunk and conjunctives. Marked hepatomegaly, 5.5 cm below the costal margin (mamilar line), of a marked consistency and a small spleen pole of 2 cm.

Laboratory Examinations

Blood: Bilirubinemia, 7 mg%, all direct. Alkaline phosphatase, 22 BU. Transaminases: GO, 180 U; GP, 900 U. Cholesterine, 4.20 g%. Blood: no anemia, leukocytes 19,800/mm³. Leukocytic formula: segmented, 13%; juvenile, 4%; eosinophils, 7%; lymphocytes, 69%; monocytes, 7%. Platelets, 310,000/mm³.

HAA: Investigation in mother and girl, both negative.

Urine: Bile pigments, ++; bile salts, +; urobilin, +.

Feces: Bilirubin and stercobilin, both negative.

¹³¹I-rose bengal test: Feces elimination of 4.3% at 48 h.

From several data, especially the high GP transaminase figures, with inversion of the GO/GP quotient, neonatal hepatitis with total retention was suspected. A *hepatic needle biopsy* gave a misleading result: In the small number of portal spaces obtained (six) some did not show a duct, others showed it with a dystrophic character and only in one a somewhat larger portal space with a moderate ductule-ductal hyperplasy was found. The inflammatory infiltration was slight and a giant cell transformation was observed.

Course: Treated only with hepatic protectors (nucleosids) and vitamin supplements, the girl progressively recovered from her dystrophic state, but the retentive jaundice remained unmodified.

At $3^1/_2$ months of age, an increase in the size of the liver and spleen was noted: liver, 6.5 cm, and with a harder consistency, and spleen, 3 cm.

Laboratory Examinations

Blood: Transaminases: GO, 52.9 mU/ml; GP, 34.5 mU/ml. Alkaline phosphatase, 13.2 BU. Cholesterol, 2.42 g%. Total bilirubin, 4.36 mg%; monoconjugated, 0.68 mg%; biconjugated, 2.65 mg%; free, 1.03 mg%.

Urine: Bile pigment, +; bile salts, ++; urobilin, +.

Feces: Sublimate reaction, negative for bilirubin and stercobilin. Grigaut reaction, negative for stercobilin and traces of bilirubin.

In spite of a satisfactory development and a decrease of the bilirubinemia, phosphatase, cholesterolemia and transaminases, the constant acholia and choluria suggested a continued obstruction of the ducts. The rose bengal test was repeated, with a result comparable to the previous one: 5.4% of the administered dose at 48 h.

The laparotomy revealed a pronounced hepatomegaly with a frank secondary biliary cirrhosis.

The result of the exploration of the biliary tree is comparable to that found in case 12. A rudimentary gallbladder without bile was found, with a nonpatent cystic duct that allowed only the introduction of a small amount of serum; as a result, the injection of contrast was not attempted. The lesser omentum was thickened and hardened; it was not possible to distinguish any of the structures in it. In the porta hepatis, which was also very thickened, no biliary cystic formation could be distinguished. A surgical biopsy was obtained and the incision was closed. The histological examination showed a typical hepatic image corresponding to an extrahepatic blockage: great connective hyperplasia and intense ductal-ductular proliferation, with bile thrombi in primary and secondary (septal) ducts.

Postoperative course: The girl followed a fairly eventful course: On the third day she showed signs of hepatic miopragia and a high amonihemia. Treatment with corticosteroids and arginine hydrochloride slowed the hepatic coma. Later, abundant ascites appeared, preventing the correct healing of the wall, and producing an eventration at the navel; the ascitic fluid was finally eliminated by a small fistule. The ascites became increasingly intense, making the practice of repeated paracenteses necessary. At the age of 8 months, during the course of a fever process of short duration, she died rapidly.

The necropsy, limited to the abdominal cavity, showed the secondary biliary cirrhosis liver which was observed at the operation with even more marked characteristics, and ganglia of the hepatic hilum hypertrophied.

The bile duct section showed a hepatic duct converted into a small cystic cavity, with thick bile contents, surrounded by a thickened tissue. The common bile duct was nearly all atretic; tis top showed a very reduced lumen continued in the cavity of the hepatic duct. The cystic duct was also atretic and the gallbladder showed a very reduced cavity, without bile contents.

At the porta hepatis level, and also in a central zone of the left lobe, a considerable number of cystic and polycystic cavities with bile contents were found, some of them the size of a small cherry.

Histological examination: In a great number of intrahepatic ducts of different sizes: in the primary, and especially in the secondary and tertiary ones (and also in the proliferated excretory structures) it was very easy to demonstrate the d-d-n process. Especially near the porta hepatis, many of them had become cystic cavities, containing bile. Most of them had only traces of the epithelial stratum and in some it had completely disappeared. Color plates VB and XV illustrate the histological features of this case of extrahepatic atresia confirmed by autopsy.

Case 16

F. P. T., $5^{1}/_{2}$-month-old boy, born at term on 5-13-1971, weighing 3,400 g, artificially fed. Physiological progress until the age of 15 days.

A brother aged 10 suffered epidemic hepatitis at the age of $1^{1}/_{2}$ years. A year previous, the mother had a miscarriage of 2 months, with no clearly explicit cause.

The mother received an injection of a progestagen towards the third month of pregnancy for prophylactic reasons.

At 15 days of age, pigmented urine and increasingly less colored feces were noted; at the age of 1 month, a marked jaundice of the skin and conjunctives appeared.

He continued like this until the fourth month, with no alteration of the general condition, and even with an exhuberant nutritive aspect.

At the same time, and during some days, the family observed somewhat colored stools, with obvious greenish mucosities; at the age of $5^1/_2$ months (10-29-71), he was seen by us.

The physical examination shows a well-developed, somewhat fat infant; he weighs 7,550 g and is 64.5 cm tall. He is pronouncedly icteric, has marked choluria and plastery stools. He does not scratch himself with his hands but moves his body substituting such an action; according to the parents, he has been doing this for 2 months. Hepatomegaly of 6 cm at the mamilar line level; a small spleen pole, of 1 cm, is observed.

Laboratory Examinations

Urine: Bile pigments, $++$; bile salts, $+$; urobilin, $++$.

Feces: Bilirubin and stercobilin, both negative.

Blood: Erythrocytes, 3,800,000/mm³; Hb, 75%; leukocytes, 12,000/mm³. Leukocytic formula: segmented, 23%; juvenile, 2%; eosinophils, 4%; lymphocytes, 67%; monocytes, 4%. Platelets, 320,000/mm³. Sedimentation rate, first hour, 20 mm; second hour 45 mm. Bilirubinemia, 10 mg%, totally direct. Transaminases: GO, 300 U; GP, 70 U; γ-glutamyltranspeptidase, 44 U (normal up to 30 U); leucine aminopeptidase, 16 U (normal up to 20 U); alkaline phosphatase, 25.4 BU. According to the isoenzymatic determination, most of it was hepatic cell phosphatase; almost no 'cholestasis phosphatase' was found. Total lipids, 11.01 g‰; cholesterol, 4.75 g‰.

[131]I-rose bengal test: Feces elimination of 10.6% of the administered dose after 72 h.

HAA: In child and mother, both negative.

A *hepatic needle biopsy,* practiced on 6-13-71, showed a subacute hepatic inflammation, with manifest portitis expressed by leukocytic infiltration (lymphocytes) in some Kiernan spaces. In all portal spaces, the ducts and ductules are clearly visible, in some places notably proliferated and affected, especially the former, by d-d-n.

Parenchyma with moderate transformation into giant cells; many of the hepatocytes show a clear and manifest balloonization. In most of them it is possible to demonstrate a biliary infiltration in the shape of small grains; bile thrombi in some canaliculi.

In some zones moderate bands of fibrosis, which from the portal spaces enter the lobules. Color plate XVI illustrates this picture.

Evolutive course: The good general condition of the child, after 5 months of evolution of the icteric process with total blockage (figure of radioactive rose bengal elimination compatible with extrahepatic atresia) and the needle biopsy of the liver, suggest an *atresia-inducing inflammatory disease* but without a definite image, neither of extrahepatic nor of intrahepatic atresia.

The lack of definition of the histological image after such a long time of evolution, the low figure of leucine aminopeptidase, and the very little increase of the γ-glutamyltranspeptidase are against an extrahepatic atresia. So even without precising a diagnosis an intervention was not recommended, and it was decided to await the patient's evolution with a corticosteroid treatment and cholesteramine treatment

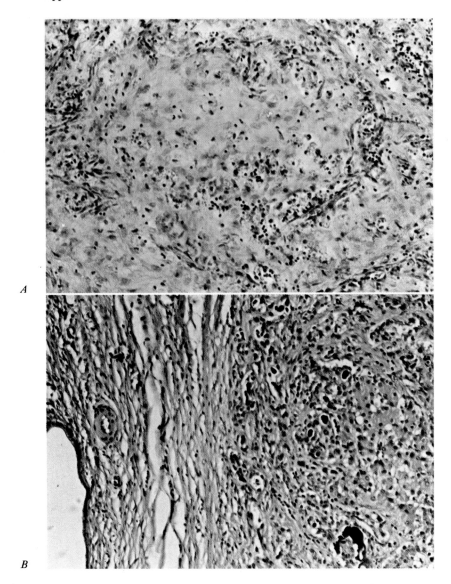

Cpl. XV. A Common bile duct lumen without epithelial traces, totally filled by a young conjunctive tissue with large and tumefact fibroblasts. Some zones show traces of bile pigment. *B* Liver and gallbladder wall. Parenchyma surrounded by an intense ductular-ductal proliferation; with many bile thrombi in the canaliculi, ductules and ducts. Gallbladder with a markedly atrophic wall. Note the flattened character of the epithelium.

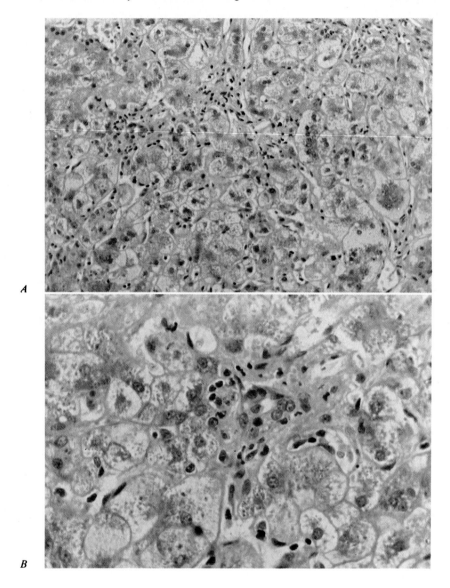

Cpl. XVI. A For a description see text (p. 230). *B* Area of the middle right part of *A* at higher magnification. Slight though clear signs of devitalization in one duct. Another duct (or ductule?) almost all necrobiotic beside it.

(predmiliden 150 mg administered during 20 days beginning with 3 mg a day and later at decreasing doses; cholestyramine, 5 g daily).

12-9-1971: Clear improvement. The child hardly shows any unusual movements and on occasions emits clear urine.

12-13-1971: Investigation of antigens associated to hepatitis – HAA in mother and child, negative. EHAA in mother, slightly +; in child, clearly +.

12-28-1971: Patent improvement of the icteric syndrome and clear decrease of the hepatomegaly; which now is only 3 cm.

Bilirubinemia; 2.5 mg%, totally direct. Transaminases: GO, 180 U; GP, 55 U.

Urine: Traces of bile pigments and urobilin and salts, negative.

Feces: Biliverdin, +; bilirubin and stercobilin, negative.

Treatment with cholesteramine and hepatic protectors continued.

1-19-72: Excellent general condition. Weight, 8,500 g. Hardly any jaundice. Clear urine, dark feces of a moderate brown color. Bilirubinemia: 2 mg%; direct, 1.5 mg%. Cholesterol, 1.30 g%$_{00}$.

2-1-72: Urine; bile pigments, negative; urobilin, some traces.

Feces: Direct bilirubin, negative; indirect bilirubin, some traces. Biliverdin, slightly +, and stercobilin, negative.

The ^{131}I-rose bengal test was repeated. A fecal elimination of 28% of the administered dose was found, discarding an extrahepatic atresia. Cholesteramine treatment, stopped.

At that moment, the differential diagnosis between intrahepatic atresia and hepatitis was undecided on account of the following analytic results:

Blood: Bilirubin, total 0.6 mg%; glucoronide, 0.4 mg%. Alkaline phosphatase, 27 BU. Transaminase, GP, 101 KU; GO, 103 KU.

A liver needle biopsy would be of great value to define the situation, but permission to perform it could not be obtained.

On 4-7-72, the dilemma was solved: the bilirubinemia was quite normal; stercobilin was found in the feces.

But it seems logical to ask: Will some traces of dysfunction due to hepatic fibrosis remain?

It is not possible to answer this question at the moment because there are some pathological blood features: cholesterol, lipoproteins and alkaline phosphatase. In the examination of 1-22-73, the blood phosphatase is still elevated (20 BU), but that of 2-13-74 is already normal. Lastly, in 11-12-74 – Transaminases: GO, 32 U; GP, 18 U; alkaline phosphatase, 17 BU. α_1-Antitrypsin, 310 mg%. So the definitive diagnosis is neonatal hepatitis and without sequelae.

Author's Index

Subject Index

– –, race and sex in 16
– –, reintervention 208
– –, remnants of ducts 67
– –, surgical treatment and perspectives of success 206
– –, total 67
– –, uncorrectable type 206, 207
–, extra-intrahepatic 205
–, intrahepatic, agenesia 127
– –, cirrhosis in 81, 196
– –, definitive diagnosis 101
– –, dysgenic etiology 156
– – etiology 156
– –, fibrosis in 195
– –, frequency 16
– –, fundamental physiopathological elements 13
– –, histopathogenesis 81
– – microscopic pathology 47
– –, neonatal hepatitis, mixed case 59
– –, obtention of a greater bile flow 208
– –, ontogenical defect 127
– –, pure (isolated) 97
– –, recanalization defect in 127
– –, zonal 14
–, preferent etiology 177
–, starting in postnatal period 175
–, total, diagnosis with greatest probabilities, nearly sure 57
–, viric disease induced *in utero* 108
Atresia-inducing, action 172
–, agent 144
–, component 189, 190
–, inflammatory process 97
–, process 66, 113
–, syndrome 190
'Atrésiante', maladie 105
'Atresying', *see* Atresia-inducing
Atrophy, disuse 14, 156
– of the ducts 14, 53, 93
– of the epithelium 93

Bile, abnormal 144
–, acids, in bile 18
– –, meconium in 123
– –, primary 18
– –, secondary 18

–, capillary vessels 45
–, duct, main, stenosis of the 97
–, ducts, direct inspection 38
– –, epithelial hyperplasia 109, 110
– –, fibroangiomatosis 175
– –, recanalization defect 109
– –, 'solid state' 109
– –, supraatresic dilation 71
–, duodenal aspiration in 25
–, elaboration 11
–, feces in 23
–, flow, obstacle to; histopathogenic expression 71
–, pigments in urine 24
–, thrombi 49, 71
Biliary stasis as a cause of inflammation 92
Bilirubin, abnormal, fetal 189
–, absorption by the intestinal wall 118
–, blood in 24
–, 'blood-digestive tract-blood' circle 117
–, conjugating system during fetal life 122
–, determination, dyazoic method 23
– –, three fractions of 14
–, direct, intestinal absorption 173
– –, passage through placenta 173
–, elimination through the intestin 112, 119
–, enteric-hepatic circle in humans 120
–, feces in, in atresia 23
–, fetal dynamics 114
–, hepatic secretion 117
–, intestinal absorption 118, 120
– – excretion 116, 119
–, meconium, deconjugation 120
–, oral ingestion 116, 117
–, passage through placenta 116
–, umbilical vessels 116
Biliverdin in meconium 114–116
Biopsy, liver, needle, value of 37, 54
– –, surgical 37, 42, 54
Blood, chemistry 28
–, cytology 28
Bloom's theory 128
Bromosulfophthalein test 29
Byler's disease 35, 101

Canal 45
–, Hering's 44, 46